Life to the Body

Biblical Principles for Health & Healing

2nd Edition

Marci Julin

Life to the Body

Biblical Principles for Health & Healing

2nd Edition

Printed in the United States of America
ISBN: 979-8-9905751-2-7

Cover by Caleb Julin. The picture idea comes from the Old Testament ceremony of cleansing found in Leviticus 14.

Learn more information at:

Dedication

For my son, Caleb.

For the first fourteen years of your life, you lived with the daily effects of a mother who was sick and in pain. From the time you were a little tyke, you prayed for me over and over again. When the burden of pain proved more than I could bear, your compassionate prayers powerfully ministered to me.

In spite of those trying years, I am amazed and deeply thankful that our predominant memories from your childhood are happy ones. I would have given anything for you to have grown up with a healthy mother, but God in His infinite love and sovereignty has used it for good in both of our lives. You are a rare blend of strength and tenderness, born out of the crucible of the LORD's work in you through suffering.

You have my honor, thanks, and love. May what I have learned and written be a legacy for you.

Contents

Foreword

He sent out his word and healed them; he rescued them from the grave. Psalm 107:20

Do you want to be well? This question might seem ridiculous at first to one who suffers physically, but upon further consideration, not quite as clear-cut as one might think. Many want to be well but only on their terms. For instance, my grandfather had lung cancer from a life-long habit of chain smoking. I remember him having surgery multiple times to remove cancer and, each time, immediately waking up and lighting a cigarette. (Obviously, this took place in the days when hospitals allowed smoking in patients' rooms.) The last time I saw him alive, he had also developed cancer of the mouth that disfigured his face and made it difficult to eat or talk, and yet he continued to smoke. Sadly, his desire to be well only went so far as steps for treatment that did not interfere with his terms for his addiction.

The Bible also contains stories of people who wanted to be well but only on their terms. For example, Naaman, the commander of the pagan king of Aram's army and yet a leper, made a long and arduous trip, hoping to be healed by the prophet Elisha. If effort indicates a desire to be well, Naaman certainly proved himself by that trip. But did he?

He had apparently envisioned a healing scenario that met with his pride's standard of pomp and circumstance. To his dismay, though, Elisha did not agree to Naaman's request for an audience but instead sent a mere servant out with instructions for the commander to bathe seven times in a dirty river. Indignant, Naaman stormed away with his entourage in tow and would have missed being made whole, were it not for the pleas of his servants. Only when this respected soldier willingly humbled himself so that he might follow the prophet's instructions did God make Naaman well.[i]

Moving now to the New Testament, John 5 tells a remarkable story of Jesus encountering a man lying on a mat by the Pool of Bethesda. We are told little about this man, other than that he had been an invalid for thirty-eight years. Superstitions persisted that the waters of the pool of Bethesda had healing powers but only for the first one who entered the waters after an angel stirred them. The difficulty for the invalid arose in being the first to enter the pool at the right moment since many hopefuls congregated nearby. Therefore, timing was critical, as was having a way to get into the pool.

After Jesus had inquired of others nearby about the invalid's condition, he approached the man. Jesus asked of him the same simple question that I ask of you. *Do you want to get well?*[ii] The man responded with a litany of evidence that demonstrated his great desire and yet continued failure to be healed. Without ceremony, Jesus simply told the man to pick up his mat and walk, and the formerly lame man did just that. So often Jesus' ways vary greatly from man's ways.

As a formerly, chronically ill person, I know the consuming desire to be well. Like Naaman who journeyed far or the invalid who anxiously waited day after day, I would have done just about anything in my power to get well. In fact, I will later detail, to my great shame, the lengths that I did go in my attempts at getting well. However, without consciously thinking it over, I drew my line in the sand when it

---

[i] 2 Kings 5
[ii] John 5:6

came to considering anything other than purely physical solutions to my physical condition. Truth be told, I very much wanted to be well but only on my terms. If you are honest with yourself, do you recognize the same inclination in yourself?

What if you could find the answers to your health problems in the Bible? You probably would not have started reading this book if you did not consider that, at the very least, a remote possibility. Indeed, a psalmist boldly claims that healing does come from the unexpected source of God's Word. Psalm 107: 18-21 says,

They loathed all food and drew near the gates of death. Then they cried to the Lord in their trouble, and he saved them from their distress. He sent out his word and healed them; he rescued them from the grave. Let them give thanks to the Lord for his unfailing love and his wonderful deeds for mankind.

This book differs from all others on health, even Christian ones, in that its pages will attempt to unfold a comprehensive picture of biblical teaching on health, illness, and healing. In a sense, it presents a broad but detailed theology of those subjects, rather than focusing in on a narrower topic. Often, the biblical teaching matches conventional wisdom but frequently it does not. At such times, I ask you to remember that God's Word is just that--God's Word, and therefore, reliable and infallible truth. I, however, am far from infallible, and so, if any principle I address brings you pause, I encourage you to study it for yourself and ask the Holy Spirit to guide you with wisdom and understanding.

I also encourage you to picture the reading of this book as a sort of treasure hunt. Each chapter will reveal another treasure (biblical principle), which might or might not be useful to you at that particular moment. If the principle does currently apply and the Holy Spirit pricks your heart, then stop and make use of your new-found understanding by taking the necessary biblical steps. If the principle does not apply at that moment, then simply tuck the treasure away for a later time. May your desire to be well produce within you an eagerness to gain the treasures that God reveals in His Word, which lead to health and life. I promise that you will be amazed at the quantity and depth of biblical principles on health found in the Scriptures that, when applied, radically transform the physical body.

So, do you want to be well? Then erase that line in the sand and learn from the Maker of all life--the true source of health and healing.

Part 1

The Wellspring

of Life

CHAPTER 1

Discover a New Path to Health

*Your statutes are forever right; give me understanding
that I may live.* Psalm 119:144

"Get a life," the gastroenterologist emphatically stated after examining me and asking a few questions about my daily activities.

"You have got to be kidding!" my mind silently screamed in response.

I was a young, stay-at-home mom who loved what I did, except for the fact that I did it while constantly feeling sick or in pain. Apparently, the concept of actually desiring to work as a homemaker proved unfathomable to the doctor. He, therefore, hastily concluded that my digestive distresses resulted from depression because I was "stuck at home" and simply needed a "real" job. Truth be told, in the years that followed, other doctors of various specialties came to similar conclusions after running test after test, which gave names to a host of chronic conditions but no explanations. I, however, deeply resented the insinuation that my physical suffering centered in my head. I knew the symptoms were real.

I know my past health scenario is far from unusual. It seems I encounter someone every week who is suffering physically in tremendous ways. Tragically, each story, no matter how unique, progresses in the same general fashion. Very few truly get well. At best, for most, the hope for wellness is ephemeral. If the individual is fortunate enough to receive a definitive diagnosis, the outcome is generally certain: The degree of suffering will progress and can merely be managed. Doctors change medications or increase dosages every time the individual adjusts to the old one, and without fail, the individual must take more drugs to combat the side-effects of the others, etc., etc.

However, if the individual falls into the other camp--where symptoms abound, but answers do not--then the doctors' appointments and tests never end; they simply change or are repeated. The suffering person longs for relief or, if that's not possible, answers. "Just give me a name to call this," is the heart's cry. Unfortunately, the name rarely results in a solution. One illness inevitably turns into another, and so the journey through life for the chronically ill becomes one of constantly thinking about their symptoms and trying new approaches to care for their deteriorating health. The hardness of life has no measure.

I knew this journey well, for I lived it for nearly two seemingly endless decades. Those who have not walked the path of long-term sickness and pain cannot fathom the impact of unrelenting, physical suffering. It wears on an individual in a way that nothing else can, consuming the thoughts and emotions till all of life's joys and pleasures suffocate in the realization of suffering. Although the chronically ill never end their pursuit for answers and help, no matter how drastic or bizarre that help might prove to be, long-term relief remains elusive. A pill, procedure, surgery, diet, detoxifying cleanse, exercise, or any of a host of other treatments might bring a measure of improvement temporarily, but almost without fail, the symptoms return and often with new ones as well.

Why is this? Is it possible that the answers lie in more than just the biological processes to which medicine points? Does real hope for health and healing, regardless of the cause, lie in Scripture for any who will earnestly seek out the wisdom and understanding from the Creator of biology? I believe the answer is a resounding, "Yes!" I hope, by the grace of God, that this book will open a long-closed door to health and healing so that those who are ill might enter in and discover true life for the body. It is not that I intend to reveal new truth, for God's Word never changes. However, culture does change, and the focus and teachings of the church often shift in response.

My journey to gaining a Biblical perspective on health began as a result of a most unwelcome book gift in 2010. You know the kind of book, I am sure. One that a friend gives you thinking it will solve all your problems and one, therefore, that you are simply not interested in reading. After a time of ignoring the tome, I happened to rise early one Saturday morning, and with the house unusually still and quiet, I decided I owed it to my friend to at least give the massive book a try. To my surprise, it addressed many Scriptural passages on health that I had never before noticed. I thought to myself that surely the author had taken the passages out of context; so I began to look them up for myself.

Like a person in the desert, who upon finding water desperately gulps in the life-giving substance, I could not get enough of God's truth on health. I began to read the entire Bible from start to finish, looking for all of the verses related to health, illness, and healing. Hour after hour, day after day for three months I obsessively read, while highlighting and recording every related passage. Completely shocked, I discovered God has much to say on such matters!

I then spent many more months doing in-depth Bible study on the passages I found in fifty-two of the sixty-six books of the Bible. That is a staggering seventy-nine percent of the books of the Bible! These passages speak directly to illness and reveal life-transforming truths. I realized then how spot-on the prophet Hosea was when he stated, *My people perish from lack of knowledge*.[iii][iv] The knowledge I discovered in the pages of the Bible changed my life and brought true healing in my spirit, soul, and body.

[iii] Unless designated otherwise, I will use the New International Version throughout this book.
[iv] Hosea 4:6

After becoming well, so many questions filled my mind. How had I missed all of these Scriptures for so many years? Why had I never heard sermons on them or had the opportunity to attend a Sunday school class on the life-giving principles that permeate the Bible? Why did God move in my heart to seek this out, and by doing so, heal me completely of thirteen diagnosed conditions? I went from not even being able to stand long enough to brush my teeth to running miles a day--not because of some pill, surgery, cleanse, diet, or charismatic healing service, but because of the Word of God. As Psalm 107:20 says, *He sent out his word and healed them; he rescued them from the grave.* I am not special or the exception to the rule. God's people do not have to perish from lack of knowledge. The Creator's principles prove true for all who will apply them. Oh, how I long to invite you to open the door of hope found in God's life-giving Word.

Questions Worth Asking

I want to use a question-and-answer approach to revealing the biblical principles that all can learn and apply. I am passionate about God's Word and have found that reading it with a questioning mind leads to answers with substance. In fact, Solomon instructed us to do just that when we seek wisdom. Proverbs 2:3-5 says,

> *Indeed, if you call out for insight and cry aloud for understanding, and if you look for it as for silver and search for it as for hidden treasure, then you will understand the fear of the Lord and find the knowledge of God.*

Apparently, this wisdom Solomon spoke of also has an impact on health because a few verses later, he continues the thought by saying, *My son, do not forget my teaching, but keep my commands in your heart, for they will prolong your life many years.*[v]

---

[v] Proverbs 3:1-2

If you deal with illness and pain or love someone who does, then you have doubtless sought vigorously for answers from the medical establishment. If the symptoms have persisted long enough and prove significant enough, then you have likely also sought out answers from alternative medicine and/or nutrition. I imagine that you have also prayed at length about the situation. I ask you to use that same persistence applied in the past to now seek out real answers about health and healing from God's Word. Let me begin this quest for truth by asking some questions that I will then answer from Scripture during the book.

- If God is a good and loving God, why are many of His children so sick?

- Are there any spiritual causes of illness or is all illness purely physical? And, if there are spiritual causes, what are they?

- Does the Bible speak of a mind/body connection?

- Does God want His children to be well?

- If God is the Great Physician, why don't more of His children get well?

- Does God still heal people today and if so, on what basis?

- Does God sometimes use illness as a form of discipline for His children?

- Are the answers to health found in eating some God-ordained diet?

- Is there any connection between what the Bible speaks of regarding the sins of the fathers and genetically inherited diseases?

By seeking out biblical answers to these and many other questions on health and healing, you will discover the life-giving principles that the Great Physician, our loving Lord, and Savior, desires for all of His children to know.

The Path of Life

Truth from an interesting messianic psalm may serve to whet your appetite to seek out biblical answers on matters of health. In Acts 2, Peter quotes Psalm 16 and tells his listeners that God fulfilled this prophecy through Jesus. It says,

> *I have set the LORD always before me; Because he is at my right hand, I will not be shaken. Therefore, my heart is glad and my tongue rejoices: my body also will rest secure, because you will not abandon me to the grave, nor will you let your Holy One see decay. You have made known to me the path of life; you will fill me with joy in your presence, with eternal pleasures at your right hand.* (Psalm 16:8-11)

Both from the prophecy itself and from Peter's commentary in Acts 2, we understand this speaks to Jesus' resurrection from the dead and that all of those who trust in Him for salvation will also be raised from the dead. That eternal life is our hope. However, biblical prophecy often has multiple layers of truth to it. The layers can be seen in a short-term fulfillment, as well as a long-term one. Frequently, prophecy also has general truth or principles that all who heed its warnings can apply and not just the original recipients.

With that said, consider the other layers, if you will, to this prophecy abounding in personal application, beginning with the phrase, *the path of life*. Later in the book, I will discuss the passage's other phrases in detail, but for now, let us simply consider the idea of a *path of life*. What is it? Is it only referring to the journey that Christians travel to eternal life? I do not believe so, and a simple word study of the original Hebrew hints at why. The word path literally means, *a well-trodden road (lit. or fig.).*[1] The word life literally means *alive* but also encompasses many aspects of the mortal life with words such as *raw (flesh), fresh, strong, quick, running, and springing.*[2] Now if we put it all together, we understand that this phrase describes, not just a someday in heaven sort of path of life, but a highway upon which one experiences a very physical and healthful life.

Jesus said that he came that we might have abundant life (John 10:10). Do you think that refers only to eternal life? No. We have physical hope for THIS life AND the one to come. Two other New Testament passages also indicate a link between the abundant life of eternity with the more immediate blessings that godliness brings to this present life. 1 Thessalonians 5:10 says, ***He died for us so that, whether we are awake or asleep, we may live together with him.*** (The psalmist uses the figurative phrase awake or asleep to mean dead or alive.) 1 Timothy 4:8 also says, ***For physical training is of some value, but godliness has value for all things, holding promise for both the present life and the life to come.***

If such a path of abundant, physical life can be made known, would you desire to know it? God's Word contains the answers for those who seek to know them. For almost two decades I completely missed the path, but now I am simply bursting at the seams with excitement to share it with you! My heart's desire is to lead you to knowledge and understanding of God's incredible truth concerning this path of life. Psalm 13:14 says, ***The teaching of the wise is the fountain of life, turning a man from the snares of death.*** I am not wise in myself, but God's Word does say in Psalm 19:7 that God's Word makes even the simple wise.

As you read the pages of this book in the days ahead, I encourage you to make Psalm 119:144 your prayer. It says, ***Your statutes are forever right; give me understanding that I may live.***

Biblical Principle: *God's Word contains knowledge of the path of life (health).*

Call to Action: *Pray daily Psalm 119:144.* ***Your statutes are forever right; give me understanding that I may live.***

CHAPTER 2

The Health Mistake of Many

Though his disease was severe, even in his illness he did not seek
help from the Lord, but only from the physicians.
2 Chronicles 17:12b

What response do most people have in our culture when they get
sick from something that lasts for more than a few days? They go to a
medical practitioner, of course.   Unless you are of a religious
persuasion that forbids medical intervention, little thought goes into
whether to visit a physician when sick. In our enlightened society we
understand a great deal about human anatomy and disease, and surely it
would be foolish not to use the intellect God gave us to inquire from a
professional who specializes in the knowledge of medicine. Or would
it?

Because the knee-jerk reaction to illness in our culture is to seek
out physicians and medicine for answers and help, I think we need to
begin our search for biblical principles regarding health with what
God's Word has to say regarding doctors. Lest warning bells now
sound in your mind for fear of the direction I am heading, let me cut to
the chase. The Bible does NOT forbid doctors or medical remedies.

With that said, God's Word does offer a couple of contrasting and
quite compelling case studies regarding the pursuit of medical

assistance, as seen through the lives of two Old Testament kings. Through the telling of their lives in the Bible, God reveals a critical principle about seeking medical counsel that many of us disregard regularly. The trials of the kings' lives, both from enemies and illness, paint a clear picture of God's desire for all His children.

Case Study Number One

After the death of King Solomon, the nation of Israel split in two, each having a king. The books of Kings and Chronicles detail the sordid lives of the many kings of Israel and Judah. Most were evil and abandoned the law of God, but every so often one king would humbly return to the God of David with all his heart. The first case study leads us to one such remarkable king of Judah, who unfortunately escapes the notice of most Christians --King Asa.

In spite of the example of a wicked father, 1 Kings 15:11 & 14 tells us that *Asa did what was right in the eyes of the LORD and that his heart was fully committed to the LORD all his life*. As a result of this inclination towards God, the nation of Judah had peace on all sides for much of his reign, and the king successfully built up their towns and fortifications. Eventually, though, King Asa did face a test in the form of an advancing, enemy nation. What would he do? Would this godly king look to the God of Jacob for guidance and deliverance or would he do what so many kings did--whatever they or their advisers thought best? 2 Chronicles gives us the answer and a glimpse into the very heart and prayer life of a leader surrendered to his God.

> *Then Asa called to the Lord his God and said, "Lord, there is no one like you to help the powerless against the mighty. Help us, Lord our God, for we rely on you, and in your name we have come against this vast army. Lord, you are our God; do not let mere mortals prevail against you.*

Hooray! Asa passed the test with flying colors, and not surprisingly, God heard the humble entreaty and gave Asa victory over his enemies. The story then jumps ahead to King Asa's fifteenth year of reign, when he received a visit from an obscure prophet of God with an encouraging reminder to always seek after the LORD.

> *The Spirit of God came on Azariah son of Oded. He went out to meet Asa and said to him, "Listen to me, Asa and all Judah and Benjamin. The Lord is with you when you are with him. If you seek him, he will be found by you, but if you forsake him, he will forsake you. "[vi]*

The prophet's message had a tremendous impact on the king whose heart inclined towards the LORD. As a result, the king of Judah boldly made many changes in his realm. He courageously stood up against the evil pursuits of his family and the general population to destroy many of the pagan places of worship throughout the land.

Then the story suddenly jumps to the thirty-fifth year of Asa's reign when the King of Israel came against the city of Ramah in Judah. Unfortunately, this time the king of Judah did not seek the LORD his God for guidance and victory. This time he rushed ahead with what seemed to him a perfectly logical course of action--gaining help by establishing a new ally. The course chosen led to a somewhat positive ending. Now you might think that the good LORD gave the king a brain to use, and therefore, he did just what any of us have done in countless situations--evaluate the facts and make the best decision we can.

However, God apparently did not see things in quite the same light. Instead, He let King Asa know through yet another obscure prophet that God did not approve of the fact that Asa relied on others for help instead of the LORD Almighty. As a result, the prophet told the king that Judah would remain at war. None of us like to be told we made the wrong decision, and Asa proved no different. Angered by the rebuke, the king locked the prophet in prison and began to oppress the people of the land.

[vi] 2 Chronicles 15:2

Almost four more years passed, bringing us to the thirty-ninth year of King Asa's reign. This time he encountered a whole new test, and one we can all relate to--illness. The Bible does not offer any commentary on the cause of the illness but merely states the following:

> *Asa was afflicted with a disease in his feet. Though his disease was severe, even in his illness he did not seek help from the Lord, but only from the physicians. Then in the forty-first year of his reign Asa died and rested with his ancestors.*[vii]

It does not say that Asa erred by seeking help from a physician, but that his mistake rested in NOT seeking the LORD about his illness. As a result, this king, who had done so much right in his life, spent the last two years of his life suffering greatly from a disease in his feet, which eventually killed him. God had made His desires clear through the prophet so many years earlier that *The Lord is with you when you are with him. If you seek him, he will be found by you.*[viii] Whether the test was an advancing, enemy army or illness, God expected Asa to seek the LORD for help. Because the king chose instead to take what he determined to be a wise course of action, the God who created and sustains life blocked Asa's path to healing.

I find it notable that God gave Asa four years to repent from his initial sin before first afflicting him with an illness and then still another two years, once sick, to repent and seek the Lord for healing. God's patience was great. Because God does not treat us as our sins deserve, He often allows much time to pass before disciplining for sin. I fear that His patience, intended to give us an opportunity to repent of our own accord, instead causes us to fail to make the connection between our sin and the Lord's discipline.

The passage makes it clear that Asa's illness, with all its suffering that eventually led to his death, could have ended differently. What a

---

[vii] 2 Chronicles 16:12-13
[viii] 2 Chronicles 15:2

tragedy, and yet how many of us who, like King Asa, truly love the LORD and yet make the same mistake?

Case Study Number Two

Let us now consider another king who also followed the LORD with all his heart, but who chose the correct path of life when confronted with illness. King Hezekiah lived several generations after Asa but also reigned as king over the nation of Judah. He came to rule at a frightening time for the Israelites: A time when the mighty, Assyrian empire pressed continually to expand into Israelite territories. In the sixth year of Hezekiah's reign, God used the Assyrians to punish the rebellious nation of Israel by completely conquering them and carrying them off into captivity.

Like Asa, Hezekiah also descended from an extremely wicked father, who even went so far as to sacrifice some of his sons to other gods. In stark contrast, when Hezekiah first came to power at twenty-five, he set about to repair the temple and restore the worship of God Almighty according to the law of Moses. 2 Kings 18:5-7 describes the king in this way:

> *Hezekiah trusted in the Lord, the God of Israel. There was no one like him among all the kings of Judah, either before him or after him. He held fast to the Lord and did not stop following him; he kept the commands the Lord had given Moses. And the Lord was with him; he was successful in whatever he undertook.*

Eight years after conquering Samaria and scattering the people of Israel, the Assyrian king Sennacherib made his move into the land of Judah. He conquered town after town on his path to Jerusalem. Can you imagine the fear that the people of Judah must have felt, knowing they were next? And so, Hezekiah faced his first significant test.

The story that followed marks one of my favorite stories in the Old Testament. Sennacherib launched a verbal assault on the God of Jacob meant to strike fear into the hearts of the people of Jerusalem. The supreme commander of the Assyrian army boldly proclaimed the king's taunts through a letter read at the city walls so that the inhabitants could hear.   The letter arrogantly stated that no other nation's gods had thwarted King Sennacherib from any of his conquests. Furthermore, it reminded the nation of Judah that their God did not rescue the nation of Israel either.

So, what was Hezekiah to do?   Recognizing the impossibility of the situation and also greatly distressed over the mockery of God Almighty by the Assyrian king, Hezekiah went into the temple of God and laid out the distressing letter before his LORD. He then prayed, and after recounting to God the bleak facts as laid out by Sennacherib, Hezekiah ended his prayer like this: ***Now, Lord our God, deliver us from his hand, so that all the kingdoms of the earth may know that you alone, LORD, are God.***[ix] Oh, that we might respond in kind by laying out before the Almighty the facts that stand against us, and then choose to place our hope in the God of the impossible!

The God who is faithful forever then answered Hezekiah's prayer by sending the prophet Isaiah to prophesy how the LORD would completely deliver the nation of Judah from the pagan Assyrian's vast army.   True to His word, God sent the death angel to wipe out a hundred and eighty-five thousand Assyrian soldiers during the night, which caused the not so mighty Sennacherib to withdraw back home where his own son killed him.   The Jews never even lifted a finger. Hooray!   Score one for King Hezekiah and for the God in whom he placed his trust!

Time then jumps forward a bit in the life of this king of Judah, and just like with King Asa, Hezekiah faced the test of illness.   The accounts in 2 Kings 20 and Isaiah 38 tell us that the illness was deadly. Instead of turning to the physicians, the King sends for the prophet Isaiah. Sadly, though, the word of the LORD through Isaiah offered no hope or comfort. He simply stated that Hezekiah should put his affairs

---

[ix] 2 Kings 19:19

in order because he would certainly die. Without further ado, the prophet then left the king. Talk about lacking bedside manner!

In typical fashion for this king who depended wholly on God, Hezekiah turned his face to the wall and poured out his heart to the LORD; *"Remember, O LORD, how I have walked before you faithfully and with wholehearted devotion and have done what is good in your eyes." And Hezekiah wept bitterly.*[x]

Before Isaiah had even made it out of the king's palace, God directed him to go back and give Hezekiah a new message: *I have heard your prayer and seen your tears; I will heal you. On the third day from now you will go up to the temple of the Lord. I will add fifteen years to your life.*[xi] And so God did heal the king who chose to turn humbly to the Great Physician.

Conclusions from the Case Studies

Now, you might wonder why I took the time to retell the biblical accounts of the different types of tests that these two kings faced. I did so because their lives and the varied trials they encountered reflected, in a general sense, the trials of all those who desire to walk with God. Tests and trials come in many forms. What becomes apparent from the telling of the tests of the two kings of Judah was that God desired for them to seek Him first and foremost in every trial of life, regardless of its nature.

In our modern, intellectual age, we Christians only give God lip service when we face illness. What do I mean by that? Well, it is simple. So often, Christians merely tack a request for God to heal them on to what THEY already intend to do in pursuit of answers and help from the medical establishment. The vast majority of prayers from or for the ill center around requests that God would heal the individual from some physical infirmity while they have this surgery or that procedure done.

---

[x] 2 Kings 20:3
[xi] 2 Kings 20:5-6

Gone is a time of prayer and perhaps even fasting to humbly seek God's insight on one's illness through the Word (the modern equivalent of the prophets of old).[xii] Gone is the searching of one's heart, along with prayers for wisdom, guidance, and healing before proceeding with our seemingly, logical course of action. I am not encouraging anyone to avoid medical treatment, but instead to seek God first and throughout the time of illness. I am stating that perhaps the Great Physician withholds or blocks the path of healing for many today, just as He did with King Asa because we fail to seek our Maker earnestly when faced with illness.

Our culture leads us to believe that disease lies purely in the physical realm, and; therefore, the logical conclusion is to seek a physical solution. And, who knows the best physical solutions? Doctors. However, we see a vastly different picture of disease painted in the pages of the Bible. If you stick with me, I will show you many principles of health and healing that fifty-two books of the Bible contain. Time and time again Scripture reveals how God involved Himself in each case of illness in one way or another. If we are to avoid Asa's mistake, we must seek God's wisdom on our health and NOT only from the physicians.

Biblical Principle: *God desires that we diligently seek His direction regarding our health.*

Call to Action: *Consider fasting and praying for a time to seek God regarding your health.* (see Appendix H)

[xii] For more information on fasting, see Appendix H.

CHAPTER 3

My Journey to Healing
From Despair to Hope

Return to your rest, my soul, for the LORD has been good to you.
For you, LORD, have delivered me from death, my eyes from
tears, my feet from stumbling, that I may walk before the LORD in
the land of the living. Psalm 116:7-9

I have noticed, time and again, that personal testimony provides the most compelling evidence of God's power. So, before I open wide the door to biblical principles on health, I want to share with you how, by God's grace, hope for healing took root in me. I will then, in subsequent chapters, share how God brought complete and joyous healing that has remained since 2009. I do not intend for the focus of this book to be on me, but to bear witness to the power of Scripture's transforming truth, I must share my health journey.

Health can be shaped at the youngest of ages, and so I will begin my story with childhood. My earliest memory of physical problems began when, at eight years of age, I began having frequent stomach aches and recurring nightmares. Being the independent sort, I attempted to deal with the problems silently on my own and frequently availed myself of the Pepto Bismol that stood ready in the medicine cabinet.   As the days of childhood transcended into adolescence, hormones and negative health exposures upped the ante.

From an early age I desperately wanted to serve the Lord Jesus as a missionary, and so I enthusiastically went, at the young age of thirteen, on the first of five summer mission trips overseas.   Through those trips, I spent almost three months a year engrossed in spiritual disciplines, which greatly deepened my walk with my Savior. Regrettably, the trips also led to injury and multiple illnesses.

Each summer brought new physical difficulties.   First came a concussion in Spain, when a two-hundred-pound beam collapsed during our construction work and threw me, headfirst, into a pile of bricks. Not surprisingly, it failed to knock the proverbial sense into me, and so the next summer I decided to travel to a much more impoverished nation. At an orphanage in Haiti, I contracted boils from the precious orphans who desperately needed love but unfortunately abounded in skin diseases.   The boils led to a year of taking ever-stronger antibiotics in an attempt to eliminate the staph infection causing the troublesome sores. (For all those who have been fortunate enough to avoid the physical suffering of the biblical Job, you will have to trust me: Boils are excruciating!)

The other foreign exposures to parasites, heavy metal toxicity, and who knows what else came in uncertain order, but one thing was certain: my body struggled greatly by the end of my last mission trip to India at seventeen years of age.   It turns out that drinking unfiltered water will make a person quite sick! We short-sighted teenagers all learned that particular truth the hard way. Upon my return to the states, my American doctor failed to recognize and properly treat the foreign ailments, and so it would be many, many years before treatment would ensue. After the summer in India, I began to go through cycles when I could only eat plain, white rice, due to my incredible digestive distress.

I also suffered from severe menstrual cycles, and by the age of eighteen, my gynecologist felt certain that I had endometriosis. Many years later another doctor confirmed the diagnosis during surgery. Even though the pain was frequent, the cascade of health struggles had barely begun. At twenty years of age, I married the man of my dreams, but because we were both still full-time students in college, stress was high, money scarce, and my abdominal pain never seemed to end. Thanks to a friend who gave us money for the appointment, I went to see a doctor. His conclusion was simple: "You have endometriosis. Either get pregnant or have surgery."

Dreaming of a little cherub to love certainly sounded more desirable than a surgery we could not afford, so we chose the pregnancy option. Hooray! Within three months I was pregnant. Unfortunately, pregnancy did not prove to be the magic bullet I sought. Instead, it greatly exacerbated the hormone problems that caused the endometriosis in the first place, and I almost miscarried. Some most unwelcome visitors called Epstein-Barr virus and chronic fatigue syndrome also joined the scene. After a difficult pregnancy, I delivered a marvelous son, whom we named Caleb. As God would have it, Caleb would be our only child due to infertility caused by my hormonal imbalances. Nonetheless, motherhood filled my heart with contentment and joy, unlike anything I had ever known. I felt certain that it was for this purpose God had created me.

In spite of my new happiness, my body struggled continuously. I suddenly began passing out and going into convulsions when I rose too quickly from lying down. After initially being misdiagnosed with epilepsy and put on medication for a couple of years, a doctor discovered through a tilt-table test that I actually had neurocardiogenic syncope. As a result of that condition, my brain sent erroneous messages to my heart to lower my blood pressure whenever I changed positions. Normally, the opposite happens so as to keep a constant supply of blood to the brain. Because of my already low blood pressure, the brain's confusing signals to the heart caused my blood pressure to drop below forty, which produced convulsions. Increasing salt intake thankfully brought the problem under control. If only there had been such a simple solution to the almost constant abdominal pain and utter exhaustion that continued to plague me daily.

[3]As my adult years progressed so did the number of diagnoses. Through the years, doctor after doctor tried one test and recommendation after another, all to no avail. Because I am a person who thrives on activity and accomplishment, I kept going full tilt anyway for most of those years, always pushing myself through the pain. During that time, usually, only God and my family saw the hurt etched in my brow at the end of the day and heard my cries for relief. Many nights I literally woke myself up from sleep by crying because of the pain that never ended.

Once again, I began having excruciating pain after eating, but this time even a bland food diet of rice and water worsened the pain. One of these times I lost thirteen pounds in six days, as documented by the doctor who promptly placed me in the hospital for eleven days. A similar scenario occurred a second time. Even when eating was not the main problem, my hormone issues caused monthly ovarian cysts and a fibroid, which, along with the endometriosis, also caused much pain. I had three surgeries to remove endometrial tissue over the course of about seven years. Somewhere along the way, fibromyalgia also joined the ranks of the other torments. Life grew increasingly more difficult from one year to the next and with no hope in sight. I longed to die.

Then, I thought I had finally found the hope I dreamed of in the form of a knowledgeable and caring naturopathic MD. He ran a litany of hormone tests and, upon seeing the results, declared me a "hormone nightmare." He stated that in his numerous years of medical practice he had never seen anything so comprehensive or devastating as my hormone test results. Even the lab put a special note on the results to indicate that they had rerun certain tests because they could not believe the accuracy of such low numbers. For example, on a scale of 0-10, my cortisol levels, which show adrenal function, were .5 at the highest point in the day. It was as if my body was just shutting down but without explanation. Other tests led to the diagnoses of heavy metal toxicity, severe anemia, a goiter, and other thyroid deficiencies, confirming hypothyroidism.

Although you might wonder how I found hope in any of this, I most certainly did. You see, I finally had names for conditions that could be treated specifically, and those names seemed to be the root of much of my physical suffering. "Surely now I will get better," I thought. For a time, some improvement did come through extensive hormone therapy and thyroid medication. Unfortunately, although hormones were at the root of many of my conditions, something had to have caused the hormones to get so terribly out-of-whack in the first place. As so frequently occurs when you treat symptoms rather than the root of the problem, eventually my body merely compensated, and the symptoms returned. My hope proved devastatingly ephemeral, and despair rebounded with the severity of symptoms. Surprisingly, the worst was still to come.

With things already desperate, the ability to continually push myself through the suffering finally came to a screeching halt. Due to a herniated disc and pinched nerve in my neck, I sought the help of a chiropractor for the first time in 2007. Tragically, I proved too fragile for snapping and cracking, and a disc in my low back announced its injury during my first adjustment with a sound like a gun firing, followed by my piercing scream. Those who have experienced an injured disc can testify to the all-consuming nature of such pain. In more ways than one, that injury was the straw that broke the camel's back. I was officially an invalid.

Dealing with relentless pain is one thing, but being unable to feel useful or even to have fun with my family was agonizing. After all, I was young, a wife and mother, and supposed to have a lifetime ahead of me to anticipate. Instead, I dreaded the future and prayed that God would just take me.

For a solid year, I sought relief from the pain of the injured discs and pinched nerve by resting on ice or heat in a recliner by my bedroom window. Since I barely had the strength to walk or stand, that chair became my haven. God had brought me to the end of being able to distract myself with activity. During this period of seclusion and incapacitation, I had plenty of time and motivation to seek the Lord fervently. Staring out the window, hour after hour, day after day, I pleaded with the Lord for answers.

Hope Takes Root

The answers certainly did not come in the way or the time frame I longed for, but by God's incredible grace, they came, nonetheless. (Although this next part of my health journey may at first seem irrelevant, the significance of the Lord bringing healing to my heart and mind proved paramount to the healing of my body, and so I ask that you bear with me.)

With time on my hands, I decided to seek out a Christian counselor to help me address a tragedy from eight years earlier with which I had never adequately dealt. Wisely, the counselor discerned the root of my struggles even though I was unaware of it at the time. She pointed out that I did not seem to trust God's Word as true and applicable to me when it spoke words of love. Not surprisingly, I believed God's Word in the hard teachings but overlooked the countless passages in which God affirmed His love for me.

Although I had spent years suffering and searching for answers, the counselor's insight made me realize the true crux of my struggle. It went far deeper than the frequently asked question concerning WHY God allows pain. The heart of the struggle was that, because of my pain, I felt unloved by God and therefore could not trust Him. Until this central issue was resolved, all other attempts at coming to grips with my suffering became temporary fixes at best.

The revelation that I mistrusted God's heart and my counselor's challenge to search for Bible passages that speak of God's love led me to a short but powerful prayer found in Ephesians 3. With determination, I chose to trust the truth of Ephesians 3:16-21, even though I did not understand it. So began months of meditation, prayer, and contemplation on those inspired words. That prayer launched a transforming journey to understanding God's love for me when some of the events of my life indicated otherwise.

With the counselor's challenge in mind to choose to trust all of God's Word, regardless of what SEEMED true, Psalm 41:1-3 jumped out at me one day during my private devotions.

Blessed are those who have regard for the weak; the Lord delivers them in times of trouble. The Lord protects and preserves them. They are counted among the blessed in the land. He does not give them over to the desire of their foes. The Lord sustains them on their sickbed and restores them from their bed of illness.

"Wow!" I thought. "Did this apply to me?" Not to toot my own horn, but I had always had tremendous regard and mercy for the weak. According to this passage, God would not only sustain such people on their sickbeds but also restore them. In the past, I would have read quickly over that passage and assumed it was merely figurative. However, on that day I paused to consider it carefully. I felt that God was asking me if I would choose to believe this passage as a promise of His intention to heal me. To some from the "name it and claim it" manner of thinking about Scripture, believing this promise might seem a no-brainer. To me, though, it was huge! Let me explain.

Church had taught me that God uses suffering to make us more like Christ. True! I also believed as many do, that God frequently uses illness in the same manner. Therefore, if my desire was to be conformed to the likeness of Christ, then I should submit to His will, rather than asking for deliverance from it. As a result, I only prayed for God to help me bear up under the physical suffering. You know--to take up my cross and follow Him.[xiii] I thought illness was my lot in life, and God would glorify himself through my suffering. Therefore, I concluded that it would be wrong to ask God to heal me.

However, there it was before me in black and white: *The Lord sustains them on their sickbed and RESTORES them from their bed*

[xiii] Matthew 16:24

of illness.[xiv] So, after some moments of contemplation, I did choose to trust that this was what God intended to do for me. I even placed a date and notation in the margin of the passage. A tiny kernel of hope and faith sprouted in me, and by God's grace, it did grow.

Over the course of the next several months, I meditated, studied, and prayed Ephesians 3:16-21. It says,

> *I pray that out of his glorious riches he may strengthen you with power through his Spirit in your inner being, so that Christ may dwell in your hearts through faith. And I pray that you, being rooted and established in love, may have power, together with all the Lord's holy people, to grasp how wide and long and high and deep is the love of Christ, and to know this love that surpasses knowledge—that you may be filled to the measure of all the fullness of God. Now to him who is able to do immeasurably more than all we ask or imagine, according to his power that is at work within us, to him be glory in the church and in Christ Jesus throughout all generations, for ever and ever! Amen.*

Each day of praying those words, God did the impossible in my heart and mind. He filled me with the overwhelming sense that God loved me with a faithful, unconditional love, and a depth that I had never known before. Although the physical symptoms continued to announce their presence, indescribable joy filled my heart. Instead of consuming despair, I could not help singing praises to my loving Savior as I went about the house. For well over thirty years, I had tried to earn God's love, but now I had peace, glorious peace! Little did I know at the time that the hope for healing and wellness in the Scriptures centers around that one remarkable word--peace.

[xiv] Throughout this book, whenever there is an emphasis placed in a verse through underlining, bold letters, or all caps it is my doing and not a part of the original text.

CHAPTER 4

The Wellspring of Life

*Keep your heart with all vigilance, for from it flow
the springs of life.* Proverbs 4:20

Nothing generates more negative emotion in one who suffers physically than the insinuation that one's symptoms are "all in your head." This statement seems to imply or accuse someone of being a hypochondriac who fabricates illnesses and symptoms, just to get attention. Although such a condition likely exists, I suspect that the accusation rarely fits the one to whom it is directed.

Doctors especially love to label the yet to be diagnosed patient with this hurtful critique. Forgive the momentary rant, but all possibilities for illness are not ruled out by a doctor's finite understanding of the human body and limited tests. For example, as a sophomore in college, I went to the emergency room after days of frightful, abdominal pain, fearing appendicitis. Upon examination, they determined that I did not have that condition and treated me as though I was just an emotional teenager. Later, during my first surgery for endometriosis, a doctor discovered that the sticky endometrial tissue in my abdomen had trapped my appendix, fixing it in a continually bent-in-half position. When the doctor showed me the video of my surgery where he snipped my appendix free, I wanted to shout; "I knew it was my appendix!" Time and time again throughout my years of illness, I experienced similar vindication from the hurtful assumptions of the arrogant. Yes, I do understand the hurt of the "all in your head" accusation all too well.

King Solomon's perspective on health

Even so, in recent years, I have come to a new appreciation of this previously hurtful statement. The change in my thinking has greatly surprised me, but slowly came about as a result of the truth I discovered in Scripture, as well as the evidence from scientific studies on health. (I will address the scientific aspect of this in the next chapter.) Perhaps changing one word in the saying would make it a more frequently accurate statement: It's all in your *heart.* Please do not misunderstand me. I am NOT saying that the symptoms of illness, whether diagnosed or undiagnosed, are not real. They most definitely are! I AM saying that the Bible and science reveal that our heart (the center of man) has a phenomenal impact on our wellbeing--either creating health and healing or stealing life from our very cells.

The words of Proverbs 14:30 say it so well! *A heart at peace gives life to the body, but envy rots the bones.* Many of the verses in Proverbs contrast two things that are related. The verse above contrasts the two emotions of peace and envy. Both reside in a person's heart. The proverb claims that one brings life to the whole body and the other rots the bones, which contain the very source of life--marrow that produces red and white blood cells, platelets, and stem cells. Could King Solomon's statement be literal in its meaning? Now that is something to consider!

Is the Body a Machine or So Much More?

A modern view of anatomy often portrays the human body as a complex machine with the brain as the central computer that controls everything. As a result, people tend to miss the significance of verses such as Proverbs 14:30. However, as evidenced in ancient writings, scholars once viewed the heart as far more than a piece of critical machinery.   Bruce K. Waltke discusses this ancient viewpoint regarding the heart when he writes,

> *From their viewpoint, the heart was the central organ that moved the rest of the body. Ancients ate to strengthen the heart and so revive the body. Abraham offers his weary guests food so that they might "sustain their hearts" and then go on their way (Genesis 18:5). Since moderns understand the anatomy differently than the ancients, the English versions gloss the Hebrew to accommodate it to a more scientific viewpoint.*[4]

This difference in the perspective of the heart between biblical authors and modern translators produced a rather muddled, biblical portrayal of the key components of man--soul, spirit, mind, and heart. It does not help matters that great overlap occurs in the meanings of each of those words, making difficult the correct deciphering of biblical meaning.   However, going back to the original Hebrew or Greek, one discovers a staggering number of uses of the word heart (roughly nine hundred) compared with an almost complete silence about the head, mind, or brain.

In fact, most of the time when you read the word *mind* in Scripture, the original language does not reference the mind at all. Instead, it is either, soul, spirit, heart, or a generic word for the center of everything (the inward part).   Therefore, the overwhelming scriptural focus on the heart highlights its significance and should make us want to understand why God focuses so much attention on this organ.

Upon discovering the significant biblical emphasis on the heart, I spent many hours reading every one of the nine hundred passages using that word, as well as every use of spirit and soul.   What I learned in my studies explains why the heart is the foundation for the path of life, and why only pursuing medical solutions to alleviate symptoms often proves fruitless.

Unraveling the Mysteries of the Heart

Recent scientific study reveals the tremendous impact the heart has on health, but great mystery still surrounds the complexity of what was once considered a simple pump. The mystery can only be understood through the lens of the biblical teaching that within the heart resides the human soul and spirit. Just as the physical heart has chambers within that make up the whole, so also the biblical portrayal of the heart reveals chambers within--the immortal soul and spirit. Understanding that concept explains much of the confusion that comes from numerous biblical passages that use the word heart interchangeably with the words spirit and soul.[xv]

Think of the chambers of the heart as two distinct and utterly separate rooms. In one room, you have the soul, which contains all of the personality, will, desires, intellect, and all that makes the creature uniquely what it is.[5] I say "it" because animals also have souls. Your soul makes you, you, but it is purely in the realm of the flesh. 1 Peter 2:11 speaks to how temptations affect the soul by saying, *Abstain from fleshly lusts which war against the soul.*

Emotions are another component of the soul. This stands out clearly in the depiction of Jesus' agony in the Garden, knowing His time of great suffering drew near. He said, *Now my soul is troubled, and what shall I say? 'Father, save me from this hour'?*[xvi] This agony of soul shows that Jesus was fully man, and, as our great High Priest, He can effectively relate to the emotions of the soul that so often plague the human heart.

[xv] i.e., Psalm 77:6 connects the spirit and the heart as if they are one and the same. It says, *I commune with mine own <u>heart</u>: and my <u>spirit</u> made diligent search* (KJV). So also does Psalm 143:4 when it says, *Therefore my <u>spirit</u> faints within me; my <u>heart</u> within me is appalled.* (ESV).
Deuteronomy 4:9 connects the soul and the heart as if they are <u>one-and-the-same</u>. It says, *Only take care, and keep your <u>soul</u> diligently, lest you forget the things that your eyes have seen, and lest they depart from your <u>heart</u> all the days of your life.* (ESV).
[xvi] John 12:27

In the next *room* of the heart, we have the spirit. The spirit uniquely allows the potential for man to interact with God. (Animals do not have spirits.) As my husband aptly illustrates, we can think of the spirit's role like that of an electric cord on an appliance. The cord connects the device with a source of power, which, when plugged in, brings it to life. So also, the spirit of man connects man to God through the Holy Spirit, bringing life to the flesh.

A problem, however, exists within the human heart. It is divided. The soul longs for the flesh, but the spirit longs for God. A wall of division stands between the two rooms. In Psalm 86:11, the psalmist acknowledges that only the truth of God can end the division of the heart. *Teach me your way, O Lord, that I may walk in your truth; unite my heart to fear your name* (ESV).

Biblical Illustrations of the Heart

If we look back to the time of Abraham, we learn that God established a covenant of circumcision as a physical sign that would set apart the Jewish nation. This act would provide an illustration of what would happen one day, not to the flesh, but to the heart that the division between God and man might be ended. God spoke of this in Deuteronomy 30:6 when He said, *The Lord your God will circumcise your hearts and the hearts of your descendants, so that you may love him with all your heart and with all your soul, and live.*[xvii]

The idea of circumcision of the heart appears three times in Scripture. For example, Romans 9:29 says, *No, a person is a Jew who is one inwardly; and circumcision is circumcision of the heart, by the Spirit, not by the written code.*

When an individual places trust in Christ alone for salvation, God ends the division between soul and spirit by His Spirit, circumcising one's heart. Through faith in Christ, the Holy Spirit indwells the heart

---

[xvii] Ephesians 3:17, 2 Corinthians 1:21-22, and Galatians 4:6

with the presence of God.[xviii] We then have the responsibility to allow the Spirit of God to rule over our hearts, thereby bringing unity or peace within.

Since the Bible characterizes a believer as a temple of the Holy Spirit,[xix] knowing more about the tabernacle or temple described in the Bible, provides additional insight into the human heart. The original temple also contained two divided chambers. Although the larger of the two sections was the Holy Place, God chose to reside in the Most Holy Place (also called the Holy of Holies). An enormous, floor to ceiling curtain separated the two rooms.[xx] Only the High Priest could pass through the curtain into the Holy of Holies because man's sin separated people from the holy presence of God. Think of the spirit of man as the smaller chamber within the heart (the Holy of Holies) that longs to be filled with the presence of God.

At the moment of Jesus' death on the cross, God visibly demonstrated His satisfaction with the blood payment for man's sin by tearing the temple's dividing curtain in two.[xxi] The rending of the curtain symbolized that Jesus' death ended the separation between God and man. Hebrews 6:19 says, *We have this hope as an anchor for the soul, firm and secure. It enters the inner sanctuary behind the curtain, where our forerunner, Jesus, has entered on our behalf.* Because we live in the realm of the flesh, the soul desperately needs the Holy Spirit as an anchor.

In the biblical languages, the soul simply means "a breathing creature." In close similarity, the spirit means, "wind; by resemblance breath."[6] From where did this breath come? Genesis 2:7 tells us; *Then the Lord God formed a man from the dust of the ground and breathed into his nostrils the breath of life, and the man became a living being* (emphasis mine). Now, get this--the word for Holy Spirit

---

[xviii] Galatians 4:6, *Because you are his sons, God sent the Sprit of his Son into our hearts, the Spirit who calls out, "Abba, Father."*
[xix] 1 Corinthians 6:19
[xx] Exodus 26:33
[xxi] Matthew 27:51

in the Bible also means wind or breath, and one of His roles is to breathe life into lifeless creatures.[xxii] So, after God fashioned the physical body of Adam, the Spirit breathed into that man the breath of life--his spirit.[xxiii]

Therefore, from the creation until now, the very essence of life for man is found in the spirit, and that life-force resides in the heart. This is really important! The soul was present in Adam, but it was not until the Holy spirit breathed a spirit (breath) into the man that he came to life. When we understand this reality of the human make-up, we understand why it is that healing is found through the Holy Spirit. Furthermore, the source for life in every human IS THE SPIRIT within him. Because of this, if you want to be healthy, YOU MUST DEAL WITH YOUR SPIRIT. Proverbs 18:14 says, *A man's spirit will endure sickness, but a crushed spirit who can bear?*

Jesus said that He came to bring life to the full.[xxiv] If the very life-force of man resides in the heart, but it is divided, how can one have abundant life? However, when Jesus ends the division of the heart and the Holy Spirit reigns within, He breathes life into the mortal body.[xxv] How? The peace of God can calm the emotions, thoughts, attitudes, and will of the soul so that peace reigns and life flows into every cell of the body. On our own, we cannot quell the storms that war against the soul, but the Spirit dwelling in us can, thereby producing health...*even as your soul is getting along well* (3 John 1:2).

Out of the Heart Flows Life

Even though the Bible and current science do not agree on the makeup of the heart, they do agree that its state can either facilitate

---

[xxii] Psalm 104:30, John 6:63, Romans 8:11
[xxiii] Translated literally Gen.2:7 reads, *And formed Elohim Yahweh man from the dust of the ground and breathed* (#5301 to give life*) into his nostrils the breath* (#5397 spirit) *of life and became the man a living being* (#5315 soul*).
[xxiv] John 10:10
[xxv] Romans 8:11

healing or hinder it. King Solomon, the wisest man in the Bible, states this clearly and thereby, establishes our next biblical principle--**out of the heart (soul and spirit) flows life.** He says,

> *My son, be attentive to my words; incline your ear to my sayings. Let them not escape from your sight; keep them within your heart. For they are life to those who find them, and healing to all their flesh. Keep your heart with all vigilance, for from it flow the springs of life.* (Proverbs 4:20-23 ESV)

Let me break this down with examples. Suppose you are healthy but then enter a lengthy period of high stress or experience some other form of emotional upheaval such as the death of a loved one or a divorce. Such negative influences get stored in the heart where, if left unchecked, they inevitably impact the systems of your body and eventually produce illness. We see this in Proverbs where Solomon contrasts the negative impact of heartache and discouragement. *A happy heart makes the face cheerful, but heartache crushes the spirit. All the days of the oppressed are wretched, but the cheerful heart has a continual feast.*[xxvi]

Conversely, consider a condition that originated from a purely physiological cause, such as a virus or injury. The emotional condition of your heart and the thoughts it produces directly impact the body's ability to repair and rebuild itself. Again, we see this detailed in Proverbs. *A cheerful heart is good medicine, but a crushed spirit dries up the bones.* That simple verse contains so much truth, which unfortunately is lost in translation. The literal meaning of the Hebrew phrase, "good medicine," is actually "a cure." Therefore, a more literal translation would be, *A cheerful heart is a cure, but a crushed spirit dries up the bones.*

But there is more. The Hebrews used the saying *fat bones* as a phrase to depict health, which is why the Bible references the bones numerous times when speaking of health and illness. We now know

---

[xxvi] Proverbs 15:13 & 15

scientifically that marrow in bones is responsible for blood cell production, which is quite literally our life. The marrow impacts our immune system and also produces a tremendous amount of stem cells, which are foundational for regrowth and repair. So, when the verse above speaks of a cheerful heart being a cure, but a crushed spirit drying up the bones, it points to the tremendous impact of the heart on health.

Therefore, whether the state of the heart directly created circumstances by which the body is susceptible to illness or if illness came first, the thoughts and emotions that flow from the heart are directly tied to whether the heart gives life or takes it.

Making Truth Personal

As I shared in the last chapter, for many years, I suffered from innumerable physical conditions that brought tremendous suffering. All the time, I also carried with me tremendous burdens of anger, bitterness, guilt, and brokenness. My heart languished continually. Because my illnesses had medical explanations, I had no awareness that they stemmed from the life-force within me oozing its brokenness into every cell of my body. When God forced me to deal with the state of my heart by making me an invalid, He began to renew my soul and spirit with the living Word. As the merciful Savior bound up my broken heart with the balm of His truth, my body also began to heal. My story demonstrates the truth of Solomon's words to his son in Proverbs 4:20-23 about storing up wisdom in the heart because it then brings life and healing to the whole body.

People generally think the brain, not the heart, stores wisdom. Over and over and over again, though, the Bible says that understanding, thinking, and wisdom all reside in the heart. Even atheists who consider their anti-God positions to be analytical products of their brains are mistaken. God says in Psalm 14:1, *The fool says in his heart, "There is no God."*

King Solomon reiterates God's principles for health again in Proverbs 16:22 when he says, *Understanding is a wellspring of life unto him that hath it* (KJV). Our soul, with all its will, intellect, emotions, and fleshly desires desperately needs truth to direct it. Through our spirit, we can hear the truth of God, but without the Holy Spirit's guidance and rule over our hearts, we easily become deceived and soul driven. We want to believe what we want to believe! Jeremiah 17:9 says that *the heart is deceitful above all things and beyond cure. Who can understand it?*

If wisdom and understanding should reside in the heart and yet our hearts are deceitful, what do we do? The answer lies in God's Word. Hebrews 4:12 says, *For the word of God is alive and active. Sharper than any double-edged sword, it penetrates even to dividing soul and spirit, joints and marrow; it judges the thoughts and attitudes of the heart.* It was not a doctor, drug, diet, surgery, or a hundred other things that I desperately tried that made me well; it was God's Word shining the light of wisdom and understanding on the needs of my heart, which then breathed life into my whole body. We so badly want a quick-fix to our health issues, but more often than not, the quick-fix methods fail. Perhaps the reason for this lies in the need to first address the issues of the heart in the light of God's transforming Word.

So much more could be said about the biblical perspective of the heart and what to do to fix it, but the rest will come, step by step, in the remaining chapters of the book. Let me instead conclude this chapter with a prayer and a challenge. After King Solomon had completed the construction of the temple, the priests placed the ark in its new home and saw that the glory of the LORD filled the temple. With the presence of the Almighty before him and the people behind him, Solomon stood before the altar with his hands stretched out towards heaven to humbly pray on behalf of his people. He said,

Whatever disaster or disease may come, and when a prayer or plea is made by anyone among your people Israel—being aware of the afflictions of their own hearts, and spreading out their

hands toward this temple—then hear from heaven, your dwelling place. Forgive and act; deal with everyone according to all they do, since you know their hearts (for you alone know every human heart).[xxvii]

Perhaps you have read this chapter and recognize the afflictions of your heart but have never made a connection between your physical health and the state of your heart. God knows and understands it all. Look to Him and His Word for wisdom and understanding. Ask Him to make clear to you the path of life that begins in your heart. I promise you; it is a prayer He longs to answer.

Biblical Principle: *Out of the heart (soul and spirit) flows life.*

Call to Action: *Begin asking God to make clear to you the path of life, which begins in your heart.*

[xxvii] 1 Kings 8:37-39

CHAPTER 5

Scientific Discovery and the Heart

...understand with their hearts and turn, and I would heal them. Matthew 13:15

Perhaps one of the world's more bizarre murder convictions occurred following an eight-year-old girl receiving the heart of a murdered ten-year-old girl. According to prolific writer and best-selling author, Paul Pearsall, PhD, the young heart recipient began having detailed and vivid dreams of a little girl being killed. Disturbed and unsure how to help their eight-year-old daughter, the parents took her to a psychiatrist for help. After several sessions, the psychiatrist determined that the girl's dreams were most likely memories of real events and recommended that the parents contact the police.

Because the typical protocol for a heart transplant includes the sharing of information on the donor's gender, age, and cause of death, police suspected that the girl in the dreams was the heart donor. Once armed with the knowledge of specific details of the crime from the child's dreams, (such as the weapon, time, place, clothes worn by the killer, and what was said), police found and convicted the ten-year-old girl's killer.[7]

Although anonymity for the donor is standard practice, there is a method in place to connect recipients with donor families. In many cases, unexplainable changes in the recipient's personality and behavior cause recipients to seek out information about their donors. Pearsall investigated seventy-three such cases and published his findings. Each story begged the question: If the heart merely functions as a pump for blood, how can the donor's memories be transferred to the recipient through a transplant?

Fascinating scientific research in the past sixty years reveals a complexity in the physical heart that staggers the mind and confirms the biblical perspective on the heart as the "wellspring of life." The physical, emotional (soul), and spiritual (spirit) components of the heart reflect a Creator of infinite wisdom who fashioned man in His three-part image. In the last chapter, I focused on the crucial impact of the heart from a biblical perspective. After all, the Bible should be our starting place as Christians. With that as our foundation, let us consider the intriguing world of scientific research, which confirms the biblical teaching that the heart can either prevent illness or cause it. The research also confirms that the emotional state of the heart can facilitate recovery or hinder healing once sick.

Proving these claims requires the use of medical jargon and quotes from the experts. Please, do not let the technical language deter you from the simple theme found at the center of it all--the state of your heart impacts EVERY area of your health. That simple understanding provides a critical foundation or starting point on the path of life.

The Emergence of New Branches of Research

During the 1960's, a new line of scientific research emerged that considered the impact of psychology on parts of the body such as the heart and the brain. A unique and pioneering husband-and-wife team--the Laceys--led the way.[8] Born in 1915, John I. Lacey grew up in a century of discoveries. His original interest centered on engineering, but while still a student at Cornell University he sustained an injury on the fencing team, which left him laid up in bed. Not one to idly waste time, John used the downtime for reading on new subjects. Branching out from his studies as an engineering student, he found fresh interests in books on psychology and biology. Mr. Lacey's biographers indicate that a new passion resulted from those readings, which eventually led to a change in career direction.[9] After a time serving in the military during World War II, John and his wife, Beatrice (known as Bea), led the way for a new branch of science, known as psychophysiology.

At that time the Laceys asked novel questions that still interest us today and which guided their meticulous experiments and studies for thirty years.

- *Why do some individuals become ill while others do not when exposed to similar pathogens and situations?*

- *Why are some individuals more or less resilient to the effects of psychological stress?*[10]

Have you ever noticed how people often respond with great differences to the same exact surgery, procedure, diet, or drug? One person recovers from major surgery in a fraction of the time as another. One individual with stage four cancer somehow survives, while another dies quickly. Biological factors certainly play into this, but the Laceys suspected and proved that one's emotional state has a tremendous impact on one's physiological response.

The Heart Affects the Autonomic Nervous System

While the Laceys research sought to answer questions about the manner in which psychology intersects with physiology, another related branch of science developed, called neurocardiology, which sought to understand the interplay between the heart and the brain. Much overlap in research was discovered, and the knowledge gleaned from these branches of science revealed a fascinating intersection between the heart, the brain, and the autonomic nervous system. In order to understand the answers to the Laceys questions about the resilience of some in health, consider the facts that follow from both psychophysiology and neurocardiology.

The heart impacts total health through the autonomic nervous system (ANS). Based on incoming messages to the ANS, all subconscious or automatic processes of the body are controlled. This includes digestion, metabolism, heart rate, blood pressure, kidney function, sexual arousal, body temperature, and countless other bodily processes. Clearly, the ANS is a critical force in the body. With that crucial nature in mind, consider this: Since the autonomic nervous system controls so many vital aspects of physiology, whatever influences the ANS will have far-reaching power to impact the overall health of the body.

If you are like most people, you probably assume that if something wields power over the autonomic nervous system, it must be the mighty brain. After all, we have been led to believe in the brain's status as the control tower of the human body. However, the Lacey's clinical research revealed the brain takes a back seat to the heart when it comes to the ANS. They discovered a nerve pathway, called the vagus nerve, as well as other means by which the heart can either hold back or aid the brain's electrical activity.

Nerve pathways run up and down through the spinal column and vagus nerve between the heart and the brain. Think of the vagus nerve as a major interstate that allows for the transport of neural information between the brain and the abdomen. Some lanes (fibers) go north, and some go south. (The medical term for the nerves traveling from the heart toward the brain is *afferent*, whereas the term for the nerves traveling from the brain to the heart is *efferent*.) All along the way, the vagus nerve has exit ramps to other highways so that information can quickly travel from the brain to the other parts of the body.

How neural information travels from the brain to the heart has been known and accepted for some time, but while the Lacey team continued their research, neurocardiologists observed something radical. More fibers in the vagus nerve are related to the cardiovascular system than to any other organ. Additionally, 85%-90% of all nerve fibers making up the vagus nerve are afferent, which means that the heart sends FAR more information to the brain than the brain sends to the heart.[11]   In other words, the heart primarily influences and directs the brain, not the other way around!

The Heart Affects the Autonomic Nervous System

Research continued for almost three decades before a neuroradiologist, Dr. J. Andrew Armour, made another remarkable breakthrough—a little brain in the heart! This *heart-brain*, as he first called it in 1991, contains 40,000 neurons, as well as a network of the same neurological components that make up the brain in the head. In other words, the heart has its own, independent central nervous system, which is undeniably seen every time a surgeon performs a heart transplant. Professor Salem from Harvard explains this phenomenon:

> *Normally, the heart communicates with the brain via nerve fibres running through the vagus nerve and the spinal column. In a heart transplant, these nerve connections do not reconnect for an extended period of time; in the meantime, the transplanted heart is able to function in its new host only through the capacity of its intact, intrinsic nervous system.*[12]

Cardiologists also observed an unexplained set of afferent nerves that looped back to the heart rather than continuing on to the brain. Remarkably, these mysterious looped nerve fibers headed back to the little brain in the heart providing a sort of thermostat or control system for the heart.[13] Medical science once assumed that the brain took care of all of the neural processing of information, but with the discovery of the heart-brain, a different picture of body function emerged. The heart-brain may be small, but the great Engineer and Creator of all designed a complex system to self-regulate the heart and to greatly influence the autonomic nervous system!

Everyone constantly experiences the impact of the heart-brain on the ANS. Have you ever gone to the doctor's office and had your blood pressure increase from the anxiety of being there? Or perhaps you have experienced the common complaint of becoming constipated or having episodes of diarrhea during a time of stress? The simple explanation for these and other stress-related symptoms are that the heart-brain sends messages about your fear, anxiety, etc. to the parts of the brain that, in turn, stimulate the ANS and, voila; the automatic functions like digestion or blood pressure respond accordingly. Although in most instances the brain directly messages the ANS, the heart initially kicks the brain into gear, and furthermore; without having to wait for a signal from the brain, the heart immediately responds to changes in the environment that require adjustments to heart function.[14] This is God's brilliant design of the heart-brain control system and sheds light on the words of King Solomon about the heart-- *for from it flow the springs of life.*[xxviii]

HRV as a measure for health

Heart rate variability is another topic worthy of consideration as we seek to understand the answers to the Lacey's original questions about the variations between individuals to illness and their resilience when stressed. When your blood pressure is taken, you also learn your heart rate, which is how many times a minute the heart beats. What you may not realize is that those beats vary in time from one beat to the next. That slight variation between beats, known as heart rate variability (HRV) provides a window into how well the autonomic nervous system is functioning. The heart brain responds almost instantaneously to both internal and external stimuli, by sending messages to the ANS to adjust your heart rate accordingly. How quickly that response occurs can be seen in the slight variations in HRV. The greater the variation, the healthier you are because it shows that your body is responding rapidly to ever-changing conditions. *High HRV is associated with healthy condition, while low HRV is associated*

[xxviii] Proverbs 4:23 ESV

with pathological conditions. The HRV is influenced by various variables such as; pathological, physiological, psychological, environmental factors, lifestyle factors, and genetic factors, etc.[15]

Of that list, let us focus on the psychological and genetic factors, which are individually important but can, surprisingly, be linked. Heart rate variability reveals the impact on your overall health as the heart responds to your thoughts and emotions through the ANS. Research shows that anxiety disorders, major depression, and stressful circumstances all decrease HRV.

Furthermore, *the impact of the hereditary factors on HRV is considered higher under psychological stress.*[16] Thanks to genetic testing, many know and fret over their genetic markers for various diseases. But what many do not understand is that just because you have the genetic marker does not mean the gene is expressed or has to be expressed. Epigenetics are the control switches that can turn the expression of those genes on or off. (I will discuss epigenetics in greater length in chapter 20.) Along with all of the emotions that arise when under stress, genetic expression also increases. Again, we see that the state of your heart emotionally mirrors the state of your physical heart and impacts the health of the whole body.

Emotions and the Heart

Many interesting studies have been done that reveal the powerful effects of emotions, both positive and negative, on the heart. One surprising study sought to determine if emotional stress was only a first world problem, but discovered it is not. One would think that those in third world countries, who daily deal with basic survival issues, would find those to be the greatest influences on their health. Instead, the study found that the impact on health by emotions was *stronger than the relative impact of hunger, homelessness, and threats to safety.*[17]

Cardiologist Dr. Micheal Miller writes about the profound influence stress has on the heart. He tells of a study *of more than*

135,000 men and women in Sweden that found a history of stress-related disorders, such as post-traumatic stress syndrome, increased the risk of cardiovascular disease by more than 60 percent within just the first year of diagnosis. He goes on to write, *On another level, we have come to appreciate that chronic psychosocial or mental stress accelerates cardiovascular disease by promoting inflammation, oxidative stress, and abnormal function of the endothelium, the protective inner lining of our blood vessels.*[18]

A massive study of roughly 30,000 individuals from 52 countries and representing every inhabited continent sought to determine the risk factors associated with myocardial infarction (heart attack). It revealed the percentages of risk for things like *smoking, a history of hypertension, diabetes, abdominal obesity, psychosocial factors, daily consumption of fruits and vegetables, regular alcohol consumption, and regular physical activity.*[19] Would you care to guess the two greatest risk factors identified? Current and former smoking topped the list at 35.7 % with psychosocial factors surprisingly close behind with 32.5%. All other factors fell far lower on the totem pole.[20] How we think and feel has a tremendous impact on heart health!

The Heart and Hormones

Did you know the heart itself produces a number of hormones? Not only do the heart and brain communicate neurologically, but we also now know they communicate biochemically through the hormones the heart produces and secretes. Many people have a general understanding of the crucial role neurotransmitters (hormones such as norepinephrine, epinephrine, dopamine, and oxytocin) play in brain activity, but most assume that all of these important hormones come only from the brain itself. This is not the case.[21]

In 1983, scientists discovered that, in addition to the heart's production of neurotransmitters, it also produces a balancing hormone completely unique to itself. This critical hormone has some unwieldy names, of which I will use the simplest--atrial peptide (ATP). This amazing hormone affects numerous body functions such as balancing blood vessels, kidney function, the adrenal glands, as well as regulatory centers in the brain.[22] The ATP released by the heart increases the release of stress hormones, which demonstrates another tie between stress, the heart, and the body. Remarkably, ATP even appears to affect the immune system.[23]

Without getting bogged down in the complexity of each part of the brain, let me just zero in on two of those parts (first the hypothalamus and then the amygdala) to highlight more unexpected ways the heart influences the whole body. Since every woman knows the importance of balanced hormones and the suffering that comes when they get out of whack, I will start with the hypothalamus. This small, but mighty, almond-sized portion in the center of the brain functions as the link between the endocrine system and the nervous system. It attempts to keep the body in a state of homeostasis.[24]

Two sources of information pass through the hypothalamus, which result in the triggering of both the ANS and endocrine glands— neural messages and hormones in the blood. *The hypothalamus has extensive afferent and efferent connections to several areas of the nervous system and the rest of the body through two major routes: neural connections and via the bloodstream.*[25] (Remember, afferent nerves are those coming from the heart to the brain.) According to Endocrine Web,

> *The hypothalamus is arguably the most essential of the endocrine system. By alerting the pituitary gland to release certain hormones to the rest of the endocrine system, the hypothalamus ensures that the internal processes of your body are balanced and working as they should.*[26]

Studies show that thoughts, emotions, and stress cause the heart to send out afferent neural information to the brain, including the hypothalamus, which, in turn, seeks to maintain homeostasis by regulating the ANS and the hormonal system.[27] This triggering of the endocrine system results in hormonal changes.

So, if your hormones, in particular, create misery for you, you have a strong indicator that your heart needs attention. Please, do not dismiss this! Hormone supplementation may be a band-aid approach to a heart issue. Now granted, changes in life such as pregnancy, menstruation, and menopause, as well as other conditions, will also cause changes in hormones. However, based on research showing the impact of the heart on hormones, the severity of symptoms of hormone imbalance, even at those times, may stem more from an individual's heart than anything.

As I have previously shared, I know first-hand the phenomenal impact that thoughts and emotions have on the body, and the havoc they wreak on the hormonal system. After the doctor declared me the worst case he had ever seen for hormone imbalances, I began taking a large assortment of prescription and compounded hormones in an attempt to cover all the bases. Taking those hormones helped me somewhat for a time, but the problems continued. I did not know for years that the root issue causing my severe hormone imbalance was my hurting heart. Oh, how it grieves me to learn of others suffering endlessly from hormonal issues. A better way--a path of life--does exist, and it begins with the heart.

Past emotional stress

What makes a particular situation stressful varies from one person to the next. To me, riding a roller coaster is great fun, but to many people, even the thought of doing a high-speed drop or loop strikes tremendous fear into their hearts. The degree of stress experienced or lack thereof has much to do with our emotional response to a particular situation.

Closely connected to the hypothalamus is another very small but powerful part of the brain called the amygdala. These two parts of the brain trigger physiological responses whenever we encounter a stimulus from our environment. However, the amygdala specifically compares stored emotional memories with the incoming environmental information from the senses. It then instantaneously determines the perceived threat level and causes the body to respond accordingly.

For example, when an abused child instantly raises his arm to protect his face every time someone lifts a hand near him, the amygdala is at work. When you smell apple pie, and your whole body relaxes because of the stored memory of your loving grandmother's apple pie, the amygdala also triggered that physiological response. When I miss my turn while driving, my amygdala triggers my heart to race and general panic to ensue because it processes the emotional memory linked to when I missed my turn to Ashville, NC and almost ended up in Nashville, TN. (Or it could be remembering the time I got lost for two hours at night while making a twenty-minute trip home from the mall. Who knows? The memories to choose from are numerous!)

The point being that not only do our current emotions affect our health but so do our emotional memories. The intricate connections between the heart, the hypothalamus, and the amygdala result in the stimulation of the autonomic nervous system and endocrine system. These responses occur before we even have time to think about them, but the more we feed and water those thoughts and emotions, the more pronounced they become as influencers of our health.

Tying It All Together

Although there still remains much to learn about the marvelous heart God designed, scientific research has revealed many answers to the questions the Laceys set out to explore. Some individuals become ill, and others do not when exposed to similar pathogens and situations because of the emotional state of their hearts. Individuals are more or less resilient to the physical effects of psychological stress because of the state of their hearts. We can certainly see through science the Word of God proved true –*A heart at peace gives life to the body* (Proverbs 4:30).

Some of us know all too well the miserable state of our hearts, but just need the knowledge and understanding of how this impacts our health to be motivated to address the root issue. If this proves true of you, I urge you to shift your focus from your physical symptoms to your ongoing thoughts and emotions. Begin praying that God will *heal your broken heart and bind up your wounds* (Psalm 147:3). Choose thankfulness, joy, and singing as you consciously take captive thoughts of sadness, unforgiveness, guilt, anger, bitterness, anxiousness, and fear.

If, on the other hand, you have a chronic illness but are not aware of any need in your heart, I encourage you to consider what comes out of your mouth as a mirror of your heart's true condition. Matthew 12:34 says, *For out of the abundance of the heart the mouth speaks*. Consider if any of the following scenarios apply to you:

- Do you find yourself quick to offer a critical remark or to complain?

- Do you find yourself verbally lashing out at others at the slightest provocation?

- Do you find yourself frequently talking about the wrongs others have done to you or perhaps verbally expressing your anticipation of worst-case scenarios?

- Do you tend to be like Eeyore from Winnie the Pooh and say things negatively or sadly?

These kinds of outward speech reflect the state of one's heart. Whether or not you have good reason to fit into any of the above-bulleted scenarios matters little. The devastating impact on your health will continue until the heart issue changes. Chapter seven will lay out a biblical and practical way to achieve transformation, but a Christian counselor can also be a tremendous asset.

When my son Caleb was little, sugar and caffeine affected him greatly, and so I monitored his intake closely. One night we hosted a party of some sort, and goodies of all kinds lined the bar of our kitchen throughout the evening. While I busily played hostess, Caleb had little supervision under extremely tempting circumstances. When bedtime arrived, I found him groaning in bed and holding his stomach. He readily confessed that my warnings of too much sugar causing tummy-aches now proved true in his experience.

Any time we experience symptoms, whether it is a tummy-ache or a chronic illness, the body attempts to alert us to an imbalance. In Caleb's case, sugar caused the problem. Unfortunately, too often we attribute all physical imbalances to purely physical causes. However, as we have seen through both Scripture and science, the problem frequently begins with the heart. Perhaps it is time to assess your physical condition with a fresh perspective. Continue the journey with me on the path of life as we discover in the next chapter the key signpost pointing the way for the heart.

Biblical Principle: *Out of the heart (soul and spirit) flows life (health).*

Call to Action: *Consider what comes out of your mouth as a mirror of your heart's true condition. What does the mirror reveal? Begin to pray that God will make clear to you any emotional areas that He would have you to address.*

CHAPTER 6

Peace Is a Path, Not a Pit Stop

A heart at peace gives life to the body...
Proverbs 14:30

If I honestly assess the default setting for my emotions, I will have to confess that inward turmoil best summarizes them. I constantly analyze myself, strive for excellence, and easily grow discouraged. More often than not, seriousness, rather than a happy-go-lucky disposition, characterizes me. That is not to say I regret the personality God created within me because I see great value in the positive aspects of my unique make-up. However, it does mean that I know first-hand the tremendous struggle of walking a path of inner peace and the detrimental impact on my health when I do not.

What about you? How would you describe your emotional status? Consider which words most generally describe the nature of your thoughts and feelings from day to day? Would you say that you are more happy or sad, loving or angry, peaceful or anxious, calm or upset, content or discontent, fearless or afraid, joyful or depressed, etc.?

As discussed in the last two chapters, a mountain of biblical and scientific evidence establishes the principle that out of the heart flows life. With the knowledge in mind of how our thoughts and emotions trigger the heart to send either life-giving or health-hindering signals, you can better grasp the importance of the next biblical principle--**the path of life is peace.**

Interestingly, even the word used synonymously for illness, *disease*, comes from two French words *des*, meaning *without or away* and *aise* meaning *ease*.[28] In other words, not at ease (dis-ease) or lacking peace. Aaron Antonovksy, the secular author of Unraveling The Mystery of Health: How People Manage Stress and Stay Well makes a case for a connection between health and peace when he says,

> *We are coming to understand health not as the absence of disease, but rather as the process by which individuals maintain their sense of coherence (i.e., sense that life is comprehensible, manageable, and meaningful) and ability to function in the face of changes in themselves and their relationships with their environment.*[29]

The sense of coherence that Antonovksy describes is nothing more than a fancy way of saying that an individual maintains an internal peace in spite of life's changes. The level at which one maintains that coherence, he says, directly correlates with the degree of health.

The Path of Life is Peace

Before I came across information from secular sources connecting disease with the state of one's heart, I began noticing a pattern or theme emerging from my biblical studies on health. That theme is peace-- God's golden thread woven throughout the tapestry of time. In spite of the abundant and rather varied biblical principles of health that will be discussed in the pages of this book, the thread of peace remains the anchor stitch connecting them all. If the heart is the wellspring of life, then peace is the very essence of health.

I shall take the same approach for teaching the pervasive theme of peace in health as used by Maria in The Sound of Music when teaching the Von Trapp children to sing, *Let's start at the very beginning. A very good place to start.*[xxix]   In Genesis 2, we discover that God Almighty initially created a scenario of perfect peace and harmony for Adam and Eve. Remember, sin, disease, and death had yet to enter the world. In that initial existence, they had no shame (peace with oneself), no marital strife (peace with man), and no barriers in their relationship with God (peace with God). Indeed, peace in those three areas reflects God's character as the three-in-one God of Peace,[xxx] who functions in perfect harmony.

Understanding God's design for mankind reveals how we best thrive. According to Psalm 139, God created each person fearfully and wonderfully. In that same passage, the psalmist speaks of God carefully forming the frame (body) within the womb. Just as a manufacturer of any product has a vision for product design and therefore knows how that product will function optimally, so also our Creator magnificently designed our bodies to work optimally under specific conditions. That design reflects the image of our Creator and functions best according to His original intent, revolving around a state of peace.

We see a connection between health and a soul at peace in 3 John 1:2. The apostle John says, ***Dear friend, I pray that you may enjoy good health and that all may go well with you, even as your soul is getting along well***[xxxi]. The well-being of our souls directly impacts our physical health because God created us that way. Yes, generally speaking, the Creator does desire that we should enjoy good health. However, that health comes when our bodies function according to their created design--in a state of peace. Therefore, **the path of life is peace**.

Some have argued that the body holds little importance to God. One might think that, after the fall, God's focus turned to restoring only the spirit and soul, not the body. After all, the body will return to dust.

[xxix] "Do-Re- Mi."
[xxx] Hebrews 13:20; 1 Corinthians 14:33; 1 Thessalonians 5:23
[xxxi] 3 John 1:2

However, that perspective misses the big picture. Beginning with creation and ending with the promise of the physical body's resurrection at the return of Christ,[xxxii] we see that the body rates as important as the soul and spirit to God.

All three parts of man (spirit, soul, and body) were affected by the curse, and God intends that all three parts should be sanctified and redeemed. Furthermore, 1 Thessalonians 5:23 tells us that God wishes to sanctify (make holy) the body along with the soul and spirit. Why? God is a God of peace and desires that the three primary components of every individual be unified and holy just like the Godhead. The verse says, *May God himself, the God of peace, sanctify you through and through. May your whole spirit, soul and body be kept blameless at the coming of our Lord Jesus Christ.*

Peace in Three Areas

Again and again, I see in the Bible that the vast majority of examples or teaching on disease and healing center around the theme of peace in one of three areas--peace with God, peace with oneself, or peace with others. Although I will delve into greater detail on each of these three areas in the chapters ahead, for now, I wish to give a birds-eye view by offering one sample passage for each area.

- Peace with God-- *Whoever of you loves life and desires to see many good days, keep your tongue from evil and your lips from speaking lies. Turn from evil and do good, seek peace and pursue it.* (Psalm 34:12-14)

  In other words, if you want to have a life of many good days, stay away from sin and instead walk in peace. We know that sin separates us from God and therefore, destroys the peace with Him that He desires for us.

[xxxii] 1 Corinthians 15:42

- Peace with oneself- *Be merciful to me, O LORD, for I am in distress; my eyes grow weak with sorrow, my soul and my body with grief. My life is consumed by anguish and my years by groaning; my strength fails because of my affliction and my bones grow weak.* (Psalm 31:9-10)

Put simply, personal inward distress, such as sadness, grief, and anguish cause a wide assortment of negative physical symptoms.

- Peace with others-- *My enemies say of me in malice, 'When will he die and his name perish?' Whenever one comes to see me, he speaks falsely, while his heart gathers slander; then he goes out and spreads it abroad. All my enemies whisper together against me; they imagine the worst for me, saying, 'A vile disease has beset him; he will never get up from the place where he lies.' Even my close friend, whom I trusted, he who shared my bread, has lifted up his heel against me.* (Psalm 41:5-9)

In short, the Psalmist connects the knowledge of others being angry with him and slandering his name, as well as a close friend's betrayal, with the onset of a vile disease.

Living In A World Lacking Peace

On any given day, most of us encounter continuous situations that threaten our peace in all three areas. We wake up and weigh ourselves or simply look in the mirror and self-criticism begins. Before everyone in the family exits the house, someone inevitably says something unkind or begins a disagreement that you have to table due to the shortness of time. Yippee! Something to leave your stomach churning about all day until a conversation later that evening can resurrect the morning's events. Oh, and we cannot forget: During the day we will undoubtedly learn of some world tragedy, or worse yet, one closer to home that feeds niggling doubts about God's love or character. Not to mention, we cannot possibly make it through the day without blowing it with some sin that, if not repented of quickly, leaves us lacking peace with God. Day after day, peace in the three critical areas of self, man, and God come under attack in this sin-cursed world.

If our health depends on being at peace, then what are we to do? That question alone can cause great stress about how to fix something so seemingly impossible. Do not despair! Let us move forward in considering the practical application of biblical principles of health. God's instruction through Solomon provides a good starting place when it says that we should desire wisdom and understanding above all else because they lead to peace and life. Consider his words in Proverbs 3:13-18.

> *Blessed are those who find wisdom, those who gain understanding, for she is more profitable than silver and yields better returns than gold. She is more precious than rubies; nothing you desire can compare with her. Long life is in her right hand; in her left hand are riches and honor. Her ways are pleasant ways, and all her paths are peace. She is a tree of life to those who take hold of her; those who hold her fast will be blessed.*

In this fast-food culture we live in, we have learned to expect immediate solutions. When I say that that we need peace in life to have health, we much prefer suggestions for something to take, drink, smoke, eat, or do to correct the problem. We want a quick fix! Yesterday! Drinking a glass of wine, popping a pill, using an essential oil, or going to a yoga class may temporarily calm the nerves and provide focus, but they fall abominably short of bringing lasting peace in any of the three areas where it is needed. They are like ointment and a band-aid when what is needed is heart surgery. Is that really what you want? More importantly, if the band-aid approach worked, the masses would not be crying out for solutions to their *dis-ease*.

In the Proverbs 3 passage, the wise king explains to his son and us that peace is a byproduct of understanding and wisdom. Keep in mind this advice comes from a man who tells us in great detail in the book of Ecclesiastes that he tried everything the world had to offer and declared it *meaningless*. Meaningless! As a result, Solomon's counsel indicates the need for a complete paradigm shift to our modern way of thinking. Peace is a path, not a pit-stop, of which God's wisdom and understanding become the map by which to stay the course. Furthermore, God provides the answers to finding these pleasant ways in His Word.

In Jeremiah 6:14 and16, the prophet Jeremiah condemns the priests of the day for ignoring the spiritual root of the Israelites' physical suffering:

> *They dress the wound of my people as though it were not serious. "Peace, peace," they say, when there is no peace. Stand at the crossroads and look; ask for the ancient paths, ask where the good way is, and walk in it, and you will find rest for your souls.*

I am afraid that the lack of biblical teaching on health from modern pulpits means that Jeremiah's criticism still proves true today. The time has come to follow the prophet's admonition to ask for the ancient paths, ask where the good way is, and walk in it. If we are to achieve and maintain good health, we must gain biblical wisdom and understanding of health, which centers around walking a path of peace.

What, then, is the answer to walking a path of peace? Before I introduce the biblical answers to that question, I want to briefly consider two of the popular approaches that the secular world recommends for restoring or maintaining inward peace.

The Medical Solution to a Lack of Peace

The first go-to solution these days when one lacks peace seems to be anti-anxiety drugs or antidepressants. NBC News reported in December of 2016 that one in six Americans takes some kind of psychiatric drugs—mostly antidepressants.[30] In spite of the extremely addictive nature and tremendous side-effects of such medicines, doctors prescribe them like candy. I am no expert in pharmacology, nor do I presume to know whether a particular individual should or should not take those prescription drugs. Many medical professionals make a case for the necessity of such drugs to bring emotional health to many individuals suffering from anxiety and depression. The prevailing thought is that, for some people, the benefits outweigh the negatives.

On the other hand, aside from the problematic side-effects like sexual dysfunction, weight gain, fatigue, and many others, the drugs have serious limitations over time. I first learned of the colloquial term Prozac poop-out while watching a documentary on depression. The medical term for when antidepressants such as Prozac no longer prove effective is tachyphylaxis. Dr. Jennifer Payne, director of the Women's Mood Disorders Center at The Johns Hopkins Hospital in Baltimore, said the following on the subject:

> *One of the problems with psychiatry and mood disorders, in particular, is that we don't know what the broken part [in the brain] is. We have a vague understanding of how antidepressants work, but that doesn't mean we totally understand the pharmacology. I don't think anyone can offer a complete biological explanation for why antidepressants stop working. But I will say this: There are [factors] that can influence someone to relapse.*[31]

Perhaps the source of the recurring imbalance is a lack of peace with God, man, oneself, or a combination of those three causing the heart to throw the brain's production and use of neurotransmitters out of sync. Treating the symptoms by manually altering the production or use of serotonin, rather than addressing the root of the problem compares with damming a river to control the flow of water. Such an approach works, but water will continue to flow from the source of the river and will constantly erode the riverbank as it seeks a way around the dam. In the case of anxiety and depression, the symptoms will, like a river, continue to flow unless something stops the actual source from which they flow. Until then, no drug will forever hold back the constant erosion that a heart without peace produces.

Eastern Meditation as a Solution to a Lack of Peace

Another popular secular approach to a lack of internal peace comes from the East in the form of meditation. Setting aside for a moment my personal belief in the spiritual dangers of Eastern meditation, let us simply consider the practice that has gained much popularity as a means to greater health. Meditation, very simply put, means contemplation, and requires the focusing of one's attention. In an article posted on the website *Yoga International*, Swami Rama describes non-biblical meditation and its goals in this way:

Meditation is a precise technique for resting the mind and attaining a state of consciousness that is totally different from the normal waking state. It is the means for fathoming all the levels of ourselves and finally experiencing the center of consciousness within.

In meditation, the mind is clear, relaxed, and inwardly focused. When you meditate, you are fully awake and alert, but your mind is not focused on the external world or on the events taking place around you. Meditation requires an inner state that is still and one-pointed so that the mind becomes silent. When the mind is silent and no longer distracts you, meditation deepens.

The goal of meditation is to go beyond the mind and experience our essential nature—which is described as peace, happiness, and bliss.[32]

Although Eastern and biblical meditation are similar in that they both require focused, prolonged contemplation, they are polar opposites in method. The non-biblical practice is to silence and still oneself so that all negative energy can be released. Peace through focus becomes the goal. The focus centers on temporal things such as one's breathing or a sound, but as soon as the meditation ends, nothing prevents the mind with all of its hang-ups and cares from coming rushing back unabated. A vacuum will be filled. If non-biblical meditation gives a break from the onslaught of stressors but fails to alter the thoughts and emotions that brought about the stress, anxiety, and depression in the first place, they will quickly return.

In contrast, biblical meditation requires a focus on God's Word, which renews and transforms the heart and mind because it contains intrinsic power to do those very things.[xxxiii]   Then, long after concentrated focus on biblical truth (meditation) ends, the Holy Spirit continues giving understanding and calling to mind the previously learned wisdom.

The Biblical Approach to Peace

If God created the body to function optimally in a state of peace, then surely, He offers a remedy for people living in a fallen world. Three passages highlight the need for peace and God's solution. God prophesied through the prophet Isaiah, *"Peace, peace to those far and near," says the Lord. "And I will heal them."*[xxxiv]   God's only Son became the fulfillment of that ancient prophecy. While speaking of the work of Jesus in Ephesians 2:17, notice how the Apostle Paul uses almost the same wording as Isaiah: *He came and preached peace to you who were far away and peace to those who were near.* Jesus himself said, *Peace I leave with you; my peace I give you. I do not give to you as the world gives*.[xxxv] According to the Savior, He alone is the source of peace, and He is unlike anything the world offers.

As a result, the apostles used an identical greeting at the beginning of their letters to the churches: *Grace and peace to you from God our Father and from the Lord Jesus Christ.* Take note: The apostles wrote this as a greeting to Christians who already have the grace and peace found through salvation in Jesus. Therefore, the blessing of grace and peace must refer to the continued need for grace and peace following salvation. Only through God's grace does the Holy Spirit

---

[xxxiii] Hebrews 4:12
[xxxiv] Isaiah 57:19
[xxxv] John 14:27

indwell believers, making possible daily peace that the flesh could never know otherwise. The Holy Spirit is the source of God's peace that Jesus offers, and no other practice, method, or drug can provide a true and lasting peace.

Our thoughts and emotions provide a litmus test for whether or not the flesh governs us, or the Spirit does. Paul contrasts the results of the flesh with those of the Spirit in Romans 8:6. *The mind governed by the flesh is death, but the mind governed by the Spirit is life and peace.* This verse is a simple guide, not only for our spiritual health but also for our eventual, physical health if something does not change. The world lives with a focus on the flesh, and their solutions to problems, therefore, remain in the physical realm. That is all they have available. The child of God, however, has literal, life-giving power through the Holy Spirit. If we continue reading Romans 8:9-11, Paul eloquently explains this power.

> *You, however, are not in the realm of the flesh but are in the realm of the Spirit, if indeed the Spirit of God lives in you. And if anyone does not have the Spirit of Christ, they do not belong to Christ. But if Christ is in you, then even though your body is subject to death because of sin, the Spirit gives life because of righteousness. And if the Spirit of him who raised Jesus from the dead is living in you, he who raised Christ from the dead will also give life to your mortal bodies because of his Spirit who lives in you.*

As believers in the shed blood of Christ, we have the tremendous gift of the Holy Spirit indwelling us, making true of us what is true of Christ--life and peace. The next chapter will reveal the exciting and practical truth (biblically and scientifically) of transforming ingrained patterns of thought and walking with the Spirit. For now, if your thoughts and emotions reveal that the flesh governs you, then I urge you to repent rather than to search for a secular solution to a spiritual problem. Although emotions in themselves are not sinful, choosing to hold on to negative ones and act in response to them places you outside of the path of peace on which the Spirit desires to lead you. Change course. Follow the signpost of peace. Then, the body God designed to work optimally in conditions whereby it experiences peace with God, peace with oneself, and peace with others will thrive.

Biblical Principle: *The path of life is peace.*

Call to Action: *Consider your thoughts and emotions to gain insight as to whether or not peace rules in your heart in three areas--with God, with yourself, and with others. Ask God to change any needed areas through the Holy Spirit's power dwelling in you.*

Find a Scripture passage that addresses the area in which you lack peace and begin to meditate on it.

CHAPTER 7

The Bible & Science On Transforming the Mind

If anyone is in Christ, he is a new creation; the old is gone;
behold, all things are made new! 2 Corinthians 5:17

Our one and only son had gone off to college in another state, leaving my husband and me as very young empty-nesters. A romantic getaway was in order. A friend and coworker of my husband generously offered us the free use of a cabin in the Colorado Rockies. The powdered snow clung to every surface, stacking up with exquisite beauty, covering any blemishes in the landscape with dazzling white, as far as the eye could see. During the day, we found no end to the adventures a snowy landscape offers. By evening though, the kind of pleasant exhaustion that comes from a day filled with tremendous fun called for a retreat within the log walls of our cabin and the warmth of the fireplace. The happy memories of that trip still fill my spirit with cheer.

Typical of our adventurous trips though, not every memory seemed pleasant at the time. On one of the last days of our vacation, we decided to experience the thrill of tube sledding at a nearby attraction. The place offered multiple broad, steep hills perfect for the young-at-heart to whisk down on a giant inner tube. A stiff wind and driving snow had kept anyone with any sense indoors; so, we had the hills to ourselves. After many trips down, my husband, Seth, and I decided to go down a particular hill while he videoed the exhilarating ride. Seth went first, filming all the way to the bottom. Conveniently, he came to a stop facing up the hill with a perfect view of my descent.

With the camera still rolling, the footage of what transpired remains for posterity. Although I started at the top of the steep hill, many feet away from Seth's starting point, I somehow drifted into the well-worn path that Seth, and probably countless others, had worn into the hillside while making an uncontrolled descent. Distracted by the filming, Seth failed to realize his path had become mine, and that I was rapidly headed straight for him.

With a warning scream, too late for an appropriate reaction from my stunned husband, I crashed into his tube and sailed through the air with a flip, landing upside down on my neck. Like a football player who, upon being tackled, lands with a sickening crunch and lies motionless on the field as the crowd holds its collective breath to see if he will rise, I too remained temporarily immobile. Thankfully, after a minute, I cautiously moved my limbs and slowly rose to discover I had sustained no injuries.

Sledding as an Illustration of Brain Plasticity

Since that incident and the repeated video viewings of the memory, I have been reminded of an illustration found in a fascinating book on neuroscience by Norman Doidge, MD called *The Brain That Changes Itself*. The author explains how every thought we have forms synaptic connections in the brain. Synapses are the gaps between the neurons and require various neurotransmitters to bridge the gaps. Because the neurons and synapses work as pathways for information, the brain is constantly forming new pathways or strengthening existing ones upon which information might travel more efficiently.

The more times we think a particular thought, the stronger those connections become, and the more likely it is that we will think that thought again. As a result, when we carelessly entertain thoughts whenever they come to visit, we give them much more power than we realize. To understand the nature of thoughts in the brain Doidge shares the metaphor of a snowy hillside, as first described by world-renowned neuroscientist Pascual-Leone.

The plastic brain is like a snowy hill in winter. Aspects of that hill--the slope, the rocks, the consistency of the snow--are, like our genes, a given. When we slide down on a sled, we can steer it and will end up at the bottom of the hill by following a path determined both by how we steer and the characteristics of the hill. Where exactly we will end up is hard to predict because there are so many factors in play.[33]

Pascal-Leone continues giving detail to his metaphor by describing how, after repeated trips down the hill, the sled naturally moves into the tracks previously created, thereby deepening the initial rut. He says, *It is very difficult now to get out of those tracks. And those tracks are not genetically determined anymore.*[34]

In a particular illness, there may be a purely physical cause that first set the illness in motion, such as bacteria, viruses, injury, nutritional deficiencies, genetics, etc. These causes would be the trees, boulders, or land fixtures in the snowy hillside illustration. Initially, those fixtures greatly influence the possible paths (thoughts and behaviors) down the hill. However, very quickly, those fixtures lead to patterns that revolve solely around the illness or pain. This is to be expected.

The problem becomes, though, that those thoughts of fear, obsessing over the symptoms, self-focus, depression, anger, bitterness, etc. steal our peace and therefore negatively impact our source for health (out of the heart flows life). Healing will be arrested. Even worse, though, is that as the frequent thoughts and emotions continually deepen the ruts, a detrimental, physical cascade progresses that may stem more from a lack of peace than the initial illness. Then it is, indeed, very difficult to get out of those tracks so that a heart at peace can once again flood the body with life.

Neurons that Fire Together, Wire Together

In my Colorado tubing experience, I attempted to avoid Seth's path by starting from a different location, but my sled naturally moved into the well-worn path of my many predecessors. My ignorance of the potential problem made me susceptible to drifting into danger. The result proved painful. Similarly, our thoughts can form well-worn paths in our brain that we fail to recognize as dangerous. A negative thought may begin innocently enough, but upon dwelling on it, the once unadulterated hillside of your brain is suddenly marred by a troublesome rut. Soon, even when you attempt to avoid that thought with something new, the brain naturally reverts to the familiar path, similar to how I started from a different location on the hill from Seth but soon drifted into his path.

Furthermore, if that initial thought happens to coincide with a particular activity, emotion, or sensation, then the two become linked. From that point forward, the sensory or experiential association will also cause the thought to be triggered, and vice versa, further deepening the rut. This defines a critical principle of neuroscience: *neurons that fire together, wire together.*[35]   Now, a vicious and seemingly unbreakable cycle of thought and behavior has begun.

Examples of such neural connections abound. If someone eats sweets when they get upset, then that behavior will be linked to that emotion, and before long, the slightest upset will trigger a desire for food consolation. If the sound of a doorbell once signaled the bearer of traumatic news, then the sound of the doorbell ringing will likely continue to trigger strong emotional thoughts. If eating a particular food made you sick, then eating that food in the future may trigger unpleasant thoughts and even stomach distress, even if the food itself is fine. If a big fight with your spouse caused you to think thoughts about the hopelessness of your marriage, then even a minor fight in the future will likely cause those thoughts to repeat themselves. If, as a child, a parent repeatedly told you that you could not do anything right, then as an adult those thoughts will likely return every time you make a mistake. If you frequently listen to a particular kind of music when you get depressed, then just hearing that music can make you depressed.

The truly scary reality of this principle, though, is that those connections widen continuously to related things. At this point, thoughts have a life of their own. For example, if you learn that you are sensitive to a certain strong smell or sound, then before long, you will likely develop the same symptoms to more and more smells/sounds and at much more subtle levels. I experienced the same problem with food sensitivities, which daily increased until I could not eat or drink anything without great pain ensuing. Unabated, the principle that neurons that fire together, wire together plays out by producing tentacles that entangle more and more areas of life.

I encourage you to take the first step by analyzing which of your thoughts and behaviors indicate neural connections that need to be broken and replaced by healthy patterns of thought. It might help to think through it better with pen and paper in hand. Recognizing what things have wired together in your mind proves crucial to stopping the negative expansion and restoring peace to your heart, soul, and body, and therefore, your health.

Brain Plasticity Seen in the Bible

Although neurons that fire together wire together has a devastatingly negative impact in a fallen world, the beautiful flip side is that the brain CAN be changed. Neuroscientists call this changeableness, plasticity. Understanding the nature of our brain's ever-changing wiring has far-reaching applications to countless areas of mental, emotional and physical health, to which I will make application throughout this book.

Plasticity is a concept that the Creator intricately fashioned into our biology, and the Bible tells us how to use it for our tremendous benefit. Romans 12:2 refers to the plasticity of our brains when it says, *Do not conform to the pattern of this world, but be transformed by the renewing of your mind.* Unwanted neural pathways that steal your peace and impact your health CAN BE made new (transformed). The method for transformation lies in replacing the old with new patterns of thought formed by the truth of God and empowered by the Holy Spirit. I have put this succinctly in our next biblical principle of health: **I can be transformed by the renewing of my mind by truth.**

Doidge says that even one minute of resisting a particular thought and replacing it with another begins the formation of a new pathway in the brain.[36] Meanwhile, the old pathway weakens slightly. Let me illustrate by continuing the snowy hillside analogy. Over time, even a well-worn tubing path can be filled in by fresh snow if it remains unused, thereby allowing for new pathways to instead be followed.

Another simple principle of neuroscience--*use it or lose it* further explains the impact of abandoning the former pathways and creating new ones We have all experienced the frustration of this principle at work when we try very hard to learn and retain a new skill only to quickly lose it when we fail to continue practicing it. Think of the parts of the brain as precious real estate in Manhattan. If a building is vacated because the occupant went out of business, that space will be quickly allocated for a different business. Space will not be wasted! Similarly, our brains never allow viable real estate to remain unused. As long as we strengthen the pathways, the brain continues to build and increase the areas of the brain required for that skill, process, or behavior. However, stop reinforcing the pathways, good or bad, and the brain will reallocate its resources to another process. Use it or lose it.

How quickly these physical changes in brain real estate can come to pass might surprise you. This speed was evidenced when Pascual-

Leone conducted a clinical study on the brains of people who had normal vision. He used a device that emits transcranial magnetic stimulation, or TMS, to map their brains and neural pathways before, during, and after a five-day period of continuously wearing a blindfold.

Their brain scans showed significant changes in the visual cortex within as little as two days. In layman's terms, the brains of those sighted individuals began to reorganize the part of the brain that once processed sight to process instead touch and sound. Shocked by how quickly changes in the brain occur, Pascual-Leone concluded that *massive plastic reorganizations can occur at unexpected speed.*[37]

Many similar experiments have since been done, and all show that the brain makes dramatic and rapid alterations based on the *use it or lose it* principle. Now, granted, such changes do not come easily. In the case of the sighted individuals, the brain changed within two days because all stimulus to the visual cortex had ended. Through this, we see that the more completely the current patterns end, the more rapid the change. I find the speed at which this occurs to be tremendously encouraging when considering the need to transform troublesome patterns of thought and behavior.

Three Steps to Transformation

Hopefully, all of this fascinating information has your wheels turning and ready for specific application. Based on the general principles of neuroscience, changing pathways in the brain requires three things--*a recognition of wrong thinking, a focused concentration, and something new to replace the old thoughts and behaviors.*[38] Interestingly, these ideas repeatedly crop up in the Bible as God reveals His method for using plasticity for our advantage. The terminology used in the Bible sounds less scientific and more spiritual, but you will quickly recognize the similarities between the two for breaking strongholds in our lives.

According to neuroscience, the first step to changing neural pathways is a recognition of wrong thinking. In the Bible, this would be called repentance, which shows itself first in the confession of sin to God. Have you considered the reason God commands that we confess our sins when the Bible states unequivocally that Jesus' blood already paid for all of them on the cross? I used to think that confession was all about the need for the wrongdoer to humble himself by admitting his wrong. That is only partly correct. One of the Greek words used for "repent" literally means *to think differently.*[39] So, confession provides a pivotal first step in repentance by acknowledging that one has erred. Without this thoughtful recognition, plastic change in the brain will never come to pass.

Once you have recognized the error in thinking that leads to wrong behavior, the second step to changing neural pathways is focused concentration. The biblical application of this is meditation. Before Joshua entered the Promised Land, God instructed him on this secret to success. Notice the elements requiring focused concentration in Joshua 1:8: *Keep this Book of the Law always on your lips; meditate on it day and night, so that you may be careful to do everything written in it. Then you will be prosperous and successful.*

The focused concentration required for memorizing Scripture so that it might always be on our lips pairs with around-the-clock meditation. In Joshua's case, he was about to enter a land full of enemies, while leading the cantankerous and unruly Israelite nation. Imagine the fear he must have felt following the death of Moses, whose remarkable sandals would certainly have been intimidating to fill. To conquer that overwhelming tendency towards fear, God instructs Joshua to focus his concentration day and night on God's Word. Likewise, the Psalms speak repeatedly of meditating day and night on the truth of God. Why? Focus on truth leads to change.

Before moving on to the third step, I want to point out one more thing evident in Joshua 1:8. Overcoming fear requires neuroplastic change that, in theory, anyone can do by applying the three steps I outline in this chapter. However, success comes from the Lord. It is His Word and His blessing for obedience to that Word that brings success. We have the Holy Spirit within us to breathe life into our mortal bodies as we submit to the transforming power of God's Word.

The third step to changing neural pathways in the brain coincides with the second--replace the old thoughts with new ones. Although this step could be thought of and practiced secularly through positive thinking, such thoughts lack the power that the unshakable truth of God's Word contains. As Hebrew 4:12 says, *The Word of God is alive and active*, and that is what we must meditate on with focused concentration to replace the old with the new.

The Maker of our biology knew the intricacies of neuroplastic change long before science bore witness to His design. Knowing the power of thoughts and emotions in our bodies, we should heed His instruction in Philippians 4:8. *Finally, brothers and sisters, whatever is true, whatever is noble, whatever is right, whatever is pure, whatever is lovely, whatever is admirable—if anything is excellent or praiseworthy—think about such things.*

Do you struggle with fear and anxiety or obsessions? Do you struggle with depression or perhaps anger? Do you struggle with addictions or any other sort of sinful strongholds in your life that steal your peace? We are not bound by bad habits, addictions, negative emotional responses, or wrong thinking that we currently consider fixtures in our lives. So many times, I have heard people say, "That's just the way I am." Nonsense! Others may cry, "It's genetic," or "I'm a victim," or "It's a chemical imbalance." Whether or not those labels are true matters very little. God created our brains with the never-ending capability to be renewed and transformed, AND He gives the born-again Christian the Holy Spirit to make it possible. We must stop conforming to the pattern of this world and instead live by truth.

My Lifetime Struggle with Depression

Although I will apply these truths to many specific areas in the remainder of this book, I want to demonstrate the application of the three steps to transformation with one example that has life and death ramifications. It is a condition that countless people wrestle with at some point in their lives--depression. Because **out of the heart flows life** and **the path of peace is life**, we know that depression undoubtedly impacts physical health in tremendous ways. As I discussed in the last chapter, the world's solutions to depression fall short of bringing lasting peace.

Depression. Just the word evokes in me memories of far too many episodes of tremendous darkness, sadness, and hopelessness. Yes, this affliction was mine. The cursed problem established a firm hold on me in the middle school years that prove traumatic to many. During the seventh grade, I became consumed with suicidal thoughts, held at bay only by the anticipation of my first mission trip months away. I remember thinking all day at school that I just needed to make it home, and then I could sleep. As a teenager, I discovered that I had the rare ability to direct the general content of my dreams, and so I longed for times of sleep when I could escape into a happy world.

By fifteen, I decided God must not exist, or I would not feel such constant despair, and so one evening while my parents were out, I began taking prescription pills to end my life. I had just swallowed number seven when the phone rang. To keep my brother from discovering what I was doing, in case the call happened to be for me, I answered the phone. God used that call to save my life. Although the friend on the other end had no idea what she had interrupted, nor did she say anything of consequence, I could not return to my desperate act following our good-byes. Thankfully, in the weeks ahead, God mercifully brought me back into a right relationship with Him, and for a time, the depression lifted.

However, as my health worsened through the years and physical pain ruled my life, I again fell into depression and patterns of suicidal thinking. I knew it was wrong for a Christian to despair like I did, but I seemed helpless to stop it. I just wanted to be free of the never-ending physical and emotional pain. Many would say that I should have been on an antidepressant, but in my stubbornness, I was never willing to go that route.

At some point, I changed my thoughts of suicide to prayers pleading that God would have mercy on me and just take me home to be with Him. This prayer became my private obsession. Even after God had healed me of all my physical ailments, the depressed thoughts resurfaced at times throughout the years. Thoughts of despair were such deeply ingrained patterns of thinking in me that they could be triggered by any incident that my brain had learned to associate with hopelessness. This is the nature of the principle that neurons that fire together, wire together. I knew the despair was wrong, but, nonetheless, it defined my private thoughts. I felt hopeless ever to change.

But, by God's grace, the change did come in the summer of 2015. That summer, everything in my life was going remarkably well, which is why it surprised me when just watching a documentary on depression triggered a period of severe hopelessness. Thankfully, our merciful God used that last occurrence to open my eyes to the spiritual truth that has now set me free from my lifetime battle. I wish to share those truths with you as one example of how to apply the three steps to transformation.

As a Bible teacher, I had been deeply studying Romans 6-8 to prepare a lesson series for the fall. In those incredibly practical chapters, which explain how to live the Christian life, I learned the magnitude of what it means to be dead to sin and alive in Christ. The chapters also teach what it looks like to walk according to the Spirit, not the flesh. By the grace of God, I successfully applied these truths and found victory in various areas of my life, but not with depression.

In the midst of the Bible study preparations, I watched a documentary on depression and began dwelling on my history with that affliction. Those thoughts triggered tremendous fear of its return. That was all it took for me to fall back into the old, familiar thought pathways. In short order, I became consumed with sadness and despair. Every night for weeks the tears would flow as I tried to sleep. The fact that the anguish I felt made no sense whatsoever only furthered the hopelessness. For days my thoughts vividly played out an image in my head of me hanging by my fingernails on the edge of a cliff with certain death below if I lost my grip. I greatly feared dishonoring my precious Lord if I lost my hold.

In spite of the depression, I continued my daily practice of spending significant amounts of time in God's Word and walking daily in the Florida sunshine while praying. One of those days while walking and praying, I again silently cried out in desperation to Jesus. "Rescue me! I can't hold on any longer! I can't live this way."

The response came as clear to my mind as if Jesus was right next to me speaking the words. "I have already saved you! You are a new creation IN me--no longer bound by the sin of despair. Walk in the new life I have provided. Quit believing Satan's lies."

Then the image came to mind once again of me hanging by my fingernails on the side of the cliff, only this time a new thought brought clarity. I saw that the scene in my mind was a visual deception from Satan, like one used by filmmakers in movies. Perhaps you know about the modern movie-making technique used when the producers want to portray a scene too dangerous or too difficult to film in real life? They film the scene in the safety of the movie-set with a solid green-screen backdrop. Later, the special effects team transposes the safely filmed scene onto the desired backdrop. The final result is a convincing scene where, for example, the actor might look to be hanging dangerously, when they were actually only inches from the safe ground during the filming.

While thinking of the green-screen filming technique, the image of me hanging by my fingernails on the edge of a cliff changed. Suddenly, I could see the deception. I was not dangling off a precipice! The firm ground of truth rested just below me. All I needed to do was stand upon it. Satan, the enemy who sought to destroy me, fed me with lies such as--*I would never be free of depression; I would eventually succumb to suicide; therefore, I should just give up; life proved too hard, and I was too weak and always would be.* I did not recognize those thoughts were lies and believing them a sin. They seemed so true, and I felt powerless to resist because I had bought into the belief that depression is merely a physical and perhaps even a genetic condition caused by hormones, neurotransmitters, and who knows what else. Yes, certainly those physical imbalances result in depression, but sinful patterns of thought become food for the roving lion.

The Holy Spirit began to flood my thoughts with the previously memorized truth of God's Word. *If anyone is in Christ, he is a new creation; the old is gone; behold, all things are made new!*[xxxvi] Yes, the old Marci struggled with depression, and in the flesh could not escape its hold. But, IN CHRIST I am new! Jesus died, was buried, and was raised to new life so that I too might be raised to new life IN HIM. In the words of Romans 6:6-7,

> *For we know that our old self was crucified with him so that the body ruled by sin might be done away with, that we should no longer be slaves to sin—because anyone who has died has been set free from sin.*

God's truth said that I no longer had to walk according to the flesh but could now walk according to the Spirit, whose very nature is *power, love, and a sound mind*--not fear.[xxxvii] With these thoughts in mind, I immediately confessed my wrong (sinful) thinking to the loving Savior and with a mere grain of faith began to praise and thank God for His deliverance (step 1 for neuroplastic change--**recognition of wrong thinking**).

Immediately the heavy, dark cloud that had been hovering over me for weeks vanished. I could once again see the sun. Oh, the joy that comes when we walk according to truth! Over the course of the next couple of days, I continued to allow God to transform my mind by renewing it according to His Word. I repeatedly meditated upon and quoted to myself Romans 6:6-7 (steps 2 and 3 of neuroplastic change-- **concentrated focus and replacing the old with the new**). With the constant reminders that I was a new creation in Christ and no longer

---

[xxxvi] 2 Corinthians 5:17 KJV
[xxxvii] 2 Timothy 1:7

bound by the old patterns of sin, God quickly restored peace to my heart, mind, and body.

I do not doubt that all sorts of chemical abnormalities involving neurotransmitters, hormones, and such-like were occurring in me during my times of depression. Depression, like all physical illnesses, can, after all, be measured and treated in the physical realm. Through sharing my testimony, I certainly do not wish to suggest in any way that someone alters their medical treatment for depression. I am neither a psychiatrist nor a doctor, but only a woman who wishes to share the transforming power of God.

Regardless of causes or treatments of depression or any illness, for that matter, Ephesians 6:12 reminds us that *our struggle is not against flesh and blood, but against the rulers, against the authorities, against the powers of this dark world and against the spiritual forces of evil in the heavenly realms*. As that passage continues, God only mentions one weapon by which to stand against Satan's attacks--the sword of the spirit, which is the Word of God. The world's solutions might decrease physical imbalances but cannot transform patterns of thought from health-hindering to life-giving ones. Only the power of God's truth brings repentance that leads to lasting healing.

Since my last struggle with depression, the familiar thought patterns have returned on occasion and threatened to reestablish themselves, except now I know to quickly resist the devil's lies with God's transforming truth. Thoughts have power, and I cannot allow sinful ones to stick around. I might not be able to help the initial thought that comes knocking, but I certainly can prevent it from taking up residence when I respond with the truth of God. "I am a new creation in Christ! The old is gone, behold all things are made new!" What an amazing, lasting peace has come from changing the devastating thought pathways that once ruled my life. As the apostle John said, *So if the Son sets you free, you will be free indeed!*[xxxviii]

[xxxviii] John 8:36

Just as a rapid reshaping of my brain occurred as I applied the three biblical/neuroscientific steps to transformation, so also can you be delivered from strongholds in your life. As you have read these chapters on the crucial nature of internal peace for your health, have you recognized any areas where inward turmoil rather than peace characterizes you? If so, I urge you to begin today to apply the biblical principle that you can be transformed by the renewing of your mind by truth. In Christ, you too are a new creation that is no longer a slave to the sins that have formed patterns in your life. Start right now to resist the devil with God's truth. God created your brain to be capable of change from the cradle to the grave. Allow Him to begin to form new, healthy thought patterns in your mind by the power of His Spirit and through the transforming truth of God's Word. Life will never be the same!

Biblical Principle: *I can be transformed by the renewing of my mind by truth.*

Call to Action: *Consider your thought patterns. Do any of them fail to match up with God's truth? Find verses that contradict the lies and begin to put into practice the three steps to transformation:*

1) Recognize your wrong thinking (repentance/confession).

2) Focused concentration (meditate day and night on the truth of God's Word).

3) Replace the old thoughts with the new (dwell on and quote specific verses so that your mind is renewed and transformed by God's truth)

Part 2

Sanctification

& Health

CHAPTER 8

An Old Testament Ceremony Picturing Sanctification & Healing

But for you who revere my name, the sun of righteousness will rise with healing in its rays. Malachi 4:2

While studying healing in the Scriptures, I began to notice passages that indicate Jesus accomplished two distinct works through the cross--the forgiveness of sins and the healing of disease.[xxxix] We all accept that Jesus died for our sins, but could the cross also have made provision for healing? The apostle Peter repeats a phrase from the book of Isaiah that suggests such an idea: ***by his wounds you have been healed***.[xl] I was beginning to consider whether that referred to complete healing—spirit, soul, AND body. If so, then both forgiveness and healing should be pictured clearly in the Old Testament Levitical system, which abundantly foreshadows the Messiah.

Some think of the book of Leviticus as a tiring book giving tedious detail on sacrifice after sacrifice and law after law. Yadda, yadda, yadda. If you are not a Jewish priest, and since Christians are no longer under the law, then who cares? It is easy to understand such sentiments

---

[xxxix] I will discuss several of these passages in future chapters.
[xl] 1 Peter 2:24 & Isaiah 53:5

from a surface reading of the book. However, upon realizing that every one of those tedious details pictures something to do with Jesus ending the separation sin had caused between God and man, the book comes alive. The vivid detail found in the sacrifices provided the Israelites (and us) with a powerful illustration of what was to come in Jesus, the spotless Lamb of God. St. Augustine explained this relationship between the Old and New Testaments when he said, *The new is in the old concealed; the old is in the new revealed.*[40]

Therefore, if Jesus' work at the cross included not just the atonement for sin but also a provision for healing, then the Levitical system established by God through Moses should point to both man's spiritual redemption and his physical healing. However, healing appeared to be absent. Not one to give up easily, I began to study the book of Leviticus in great detail. What I found blew me away!

A Disease Representative of Sin

Halfway into Leviticus, Moses launched into a graphically detailed description of skin conditions and mold or mildew in chapter thirteen. Notwithstanding the gross factor, God gave those instructions so that priests could determine the clean from the unclean. In our age of dermatologists and bleach, such colorful descriptions appear culturally irrelevant. However, despite our modern way of looking at skin diseases and walls that need cleaning, this section of Leviticus brims with application and pictures of Christ's work at the cross.

In chapters to come, I will show how God, in a general sense, links sin and illness throughout Scripture. However, He designated one illness, in particular, to be an outward representation of inward sin. Matthew Henry's Commentary says, *Leprosy signified, not so much sin in general as a state of sin, by which men are separated from God.*[41] This disease, with its progressive, outward decay illustrates the progressive inward decay caused by our sin. To further draw attention to the fact that leprosy represented the sin nature, every time the

Levitical law or Jesus spoke of healing leprosy, they used the word *cleansed* not *healed.*

Anyone afflicted with the dreaded disease had to go before the priest, who then used the details found in the Mosaic Law as a basis for declaring the individual "unclean" to ensure that they lived separately from all who were "clean" within the camp.[xli] The physical separation not only provided a means of quarantine, but it also served symbolically to highlight the separation that sin causes.

Recognizing leprosy (sin), provided a starting point for the priests, but what if an actual cleansing of that cursed affliction took place? To provide for such a possibility, Moses outlined in Leviticus fourteen what is arguably, the most bizarre and least understood ceremony in the entire Bible--the cleansing from infectious skin diseases. Now, please, do not let the gross name prevent you from learning the amazing beauty and application found in this ritual. After all, that is the point. Sin is disgusting, but oh, the beauty of being cleansed from it! This ceremony restores the healed leper to right fellowship with people and with God and symbolically pictures the cleansing and healing Jesus brings through the cross.

The very need for the ceremony of cleansing highlights the limitations of the Levitical system of law to adequately deal with sin, as represented by leprosy. Matthew Henry's Commentary continues on to say,

> ...*the leprosy of the soul, defiling to the conscience, and from which Christ alone can cleanse us; for herein the power of his grace infinitely transcends that of the legal priesthood, that the priest could only convict the leper (for by the law is the knowledge of sin), but Christ can cure the leper, he can take away sin. "Lord,*

[xli] Although the word found in Leviticus for leprosy can include a number of different infectious skin diseases, as well as mold, I will keep things simple by referring only to leprosy.

if thou wilt, thou canst make me clean," which was more than the *priests could do* (Matthew 8:2).[42]

An Overview of the Ceremony of Cleansing

I realize that at first glance a study of this obscure ceremony might seem out of place in a book on biblical principles of health. Stick with me though, and you will see that it firmly establishes a solid, God-ordained framework for understanding many of the principles I teach in the pages of this book. Prepare to be enthralled and encouraged!

Three different phases make up this ritual and combine elements of other Levitical ceremonies, both for sanctification and for the forgiveness of sins. The fact that God combined these various elements, along with unique ones, into a ceremony specifically tied to illness weaves a commanding picture. This tapestry made up of individual threads, woven masterfully together, forms the most complete prophetic picture God established in the Old Testament. Some threads foretell the work of the cross and salvation while others picture the need for peace with oneself, others and God. Last, but certainly not least, the overall picture foretells the provision of Christ for the forgiveness of sins and the healing of disease.

For the sake of background, you should know that, from all indications in the book of Numbers, Miriam the sister of Moses made use of this ceremony. She challenged Moses' sole authority and, by God's judgment, was struck immediately with leprosy. The ever-humble Moses prayed for Miriam, and God mercifully granted healing but required of her the separation and cleansing, which the ceremony of cleansing provided.[xlii] However, following that single instance, the ceremony remained unused until Jesus began healing lepers during his ministry.[xliii] It would appear, then, that God did not establish the

---

[xlii] Numbers 12

[xliii] *And there were many in Israel with leprosy in the time of Elisha the prophet, yet not one of them was cleansed—only Naaman the Syrian.* Luke 4:27

ceremony for practical use, but as a prophetic picture and testimony of the Messiah's work.

To unveil the intriguing but bizarre ceremony of cleansing, I have created a fictitious story, weaving the many details of Leviticus fourteen into the context of the story found in Luke 17:11-19, where Jesus healed ten lepers and then instructed them to go and present themselves to the priests. Another passage describing Jesus healing a leper (Mark 1:40-44) provides extra detail as to why Jesus instructed healed lepers to present themselves to the priests. *But go, show yourself to the priest and offer the sacrifices that Moses commanded for your cleansing, as a testimony to them."*[xliv] As the details of the ritual unfold, you will understand why this ceremony, above all others found in the Mosaic law, would provide a profound testimony to any priest whose heart desired truth.

A Story--The Lepers Find Cleansing

"I wonder when we'll see our leprosy disappear?" one man excitedly asked of his companions as he hobbled along on heavily wrapped feet.

"I don't know," replied another, "but the teacher said to show ourselves to the priests, which could only mean one thing."

Another of the ten spoke up in the muffled words of one who had long ago lost his nose to leprosy and now continually covered much of his face to deter the gnats from swarming the wound. "I know! Jesus wants us to show ourselves to the priests and undergo the ceremony of cleansing. That can only mean one thing--we'll be healed!"

Within moments, the men's elation knew no bounds when they discovered the scaly, white patches that previously marred their bodies miraculously transformed into smooth, radiantly healthy skin.

[xliv] Mark 1:44

Some days later, at the temple in Jerusalem, a senior priest pulled aside a younger one to speak of a sensitive subject. "Matthias, I have a matter for you to address. Word has come that the teacher called Jesus healed some lepers in the region of Galilee. These men have requested that a priest begin the ceremony of cleansing for them. I wish for you to travel to the leper district to investigate these claims."

"Surely there is no merit to such a report!" replied Matthias. "It's too far to travel for such ridiculous claims!"

"I know it's absurd, and yet, it is our duty nonetheless."

"Can't you send someone else? I will be unclean for seven days if they are lying; not to mention how foul that place smells!"

"Then, stand outside the entrance of the community and send for the men to come out to you. If they are not well, the sight and smell will be evidence enough. Then there will be no need to examine them, and you will remain ceremonially clean. If they appear to be well, however, you must begin the process the Torah specifies."

He continued as though talking to himself, "I never thought the day would come when the ceremony of cleansing would be necessary. No one has been healed of leprosy since the time of Elisha! What am I saying? This report can't be true!"[xlv]

Turning his full attention once again to Matthias, the priest continued, "Nonetheless, go now but keep this matter quiet. I expect a full report. We must silence the false claims the followers of Yeshua[xlvi] make about him."

[xlv] Elisha healed Naaman from leprosy in 2 Kings 5, but he was not a Jew and therefore would not have undergone the ceremony of cleansing.
[xlvi] Yeshua is the Jewish name for Jesus.

Much to his dismay, Matthias failed to find even the slightest indication of leprosy on the ten men who boldly claimed that Yeshua had healed them. So, after calling for the prescribed articles, the reluctant priest began the first phase of the ceremony for cleansing outside the city gates in the leper district. Taking one of the two live, clean birds, Matthias crushed the delicate creature by wringing off its head over a clay pot filled with fresh water. Its blood flowed out into the bowl swirling as it mixed with the water. Taking the remaining live bird, he then dipped it, along with a piece of cedar wood, scarlet thread, and hyssop into the blood and water mixture.

In solemn tones befitting a ceremony of God, the priest repeated, "You are clean," while simultaneously using the live bird and symbolic elements to sprinkle the blood and water from the bowl on one of the healed lepers. Sprinkle. "You are clean." Sprinkle. "You are clean." Over and over Matthias sprinkled the same man and chanted the same words until he had completed the seven prescribed utterances.

Hearing that emphatic statement from the priest of God the first time, the grown man began a gentle weeping. Then, as again and again, the priest repeated, "You are clean," a semblance of control faded until his companions had to support him as sobs threatened to bring him to his knees. The sound of words made precious beyond measure from years of being declared unclean by everyone, including himself, washed over his troubled soul.

Now altered by the man's response, the formerly indifferent priest also rejoiced in his spirit as he released the living bird. Rather dazed, the small creature shook off the remnants of death from the other bird and rose to fly freely across the open field. All stood transfixed as they watched the joyful sight.

In a voice that sought composure but failed, the former leper asked, "Is th-that it? Can I go back to my village and family now?"

"First you must wash your clothes," replied Matthias to the man. "Then shave off every single hair on your body and bathe with water."

At this, the men murmured among themselves about how humiliating and painful shaving EVERY part of their bodies would be.

Talking over the din of the men's discussion, Matthias regained their attention. "Mind you, don't forget to shave even your eyebrows. Afterward, you will be ceremonially clean. Only then may you once again enter the city gates. However, you may not enter your house just yet."

Perplexed, the man asked, "But when can I sleep in my bed and once again enjoy the wife of my youth?"

"On the seventh day, you must once again shave off all of the hair on your body, wash your clothes, and wash yourself. "

"Then am I free to enter my house before joining others to worship YHWH?"

With a cautionary hand raised, Matthias answered, "According to the law of Moses, you must travel to the temple in Jerusalem to present yourself before YHWH on the eighth day with two spotless male lambs. Take also three-tenths of an ephah of fine flour mixed with oil for a grain offering, along with a log of oil. I will meet you at the entrance to the temple and present you and your sacrifices to YHWH, just as Moses prescribed. Then, you may return to your home with all of your original rights and privileges."

Turning to each other to discuss the requirements laid out by the priest, the healed lepers determined to send for their families so that they might join the men as witnesses and companions for the long journey to Jerusalem.

Later, back in Jerusalem, Matthias pulled his mentor aside to report the news of the lepers' healing. "It is true! I could find no marks of leprosy on any of the ten. Their clothes still stank horribly of the illness, but their skin appeared smooth and new. All told the same story--that they went to find Yeshua and called out to him from a distance that he might have pity on them. Others verified their story by saying each of the men had lived for varying lengths of time in the leper's camp."

"Did Yeshua touch them?"

"No," Matthias replied. "They said he only told them to go and present themselves to the priest, and as they walked on their way to do so, they were healed. Only one, a Samaritan, went back to thank Yeshua personally and spoke further to him."

"How can it be possible that a mere man healed them of leprosy?" murmured the senior priest, more to himself than his protégé. "Only YHWH has ever healed someone of that cursed disease!"

Not wanting to disturb his mentor's conflicted musings, Matthias waited silently for a time before asking his questions. "I wonder if you might explain to me the meaning of the symbols used in the initial phase of the ceremony of cleansing? I know that the three symbols-- cedar wood, hyssop, and scarlet wool thread are also used to make the water of cleansing for temple use,[xlvii] but could you explain to me the meaning of all of the symbols in the ceremony?"

"We don't know why YHWH chose each one, but we believe them to be pictures of the work the Messiah will one day accomplish in permanently cleansing man from sin. Hyssop, of course, was used to place the blood over the tops and sides of our fathers' doorways so that the death angel might pass over their homes on the last night in Egypt.[xlviii] King David also speaks in the Psalms of Adonai cleansing us with hyssop so that we might be whiter than snow,[xlix] but you know all of that."

"Yes, yes," replied Matthias. "The scarlet wool is also easy, of course. It represents the blood that cleanses from sin. But what of the wood?"

"Matthias, clearly you need to spend more time studying Levitical law," the mentor commented disapprovingly. "Wood represents humanity, and YHWH commanded that anyone hung on a tree is

---

[xlvii] Numbers 19:18
[xlviii] Exodus 10:22
[xlix] Psalm 51:7

cursed by Him.[i] Although, I must admit that it is a mystery to me why Adonai would directly combine the curse of humanity with the elements of cleansing."

"Forgive me if it's improper for me to suggest a reason, but could that represent that YHWH will one day take on the flesh of man as the Messiah?"

"Some in the Sanhedrin do believe that the Messiah will be more than just a man--the actual Son of YHWH, but much debate surrounds that question.[ii] I, myself, have been undecided on the matter, although your observation from the symbols in the ceremony of cleansing gives me more to consider." With a light in his eyes, the senior priest replied, "There's hope for you yet, Matthias."

"If you please; why was I to use the blood of a bird and not a lamb?"

"That answer, my son, is a mystery. Unlike the times when YHWH allows the poor to substitute birds for livestock in certain sacrifices, this use of birds appears to have a symbolic reason rather than a practical one. All I can say is that YHWH will reveal all mysteries in the end. Ours is to watch and wait for the revealing."

"I do know what the clay pot represents, teacher. Adonai is the potter, and we are the clay, so the basin also pictures humanity, which needs cleansing."

"Very good, Matthias. That leaves only the blood and the water, which fill the pot. Clearly, they too represent cleansing from sin. As you know, YHWH instructs priests first to wash the inner parts, as well as the legs of the sacrifice with fresh water before burning all burnt

---

[i] *And if a man has committed a crime punishable by death and he is put to death, and you hang him on a tree, his body shall not remain all night on the tree, but you shall bury him the same day, for a hanged man is cursed by God.* Deuteronomy 21:22-23 (ESV)

[ii] In Luke 22:70-23:3 Jesus claims to be the Son of God while on trial before the Sanhedrin, which causes them to rush Jesus before Pilate because they equated that claim with the claim to be the Christ.

offerings before the LORD.[lii]   The pure water cleanses the sacrifice so that it might then be presented to YHWH. However, the direct mixing together of the blood and the water for sprinkling remains unique to the ceremony of cleansing and somewhat of a mystery.   They must symbolize an element unique to the work of the Messiah."

"Surely, we have much to contemplate," replied Matthias.

"What intrigues me most, my son, is that this Yeshua has made necessary a long, unused ceremony so filled with pictures of the Messiah's cleansing work. What could it possibly mean?"

On the seventh day, outside the gates of Jerusalem, the ten healed lepers again washed their bodies and clothes. Still itching fiercely all over from the shaving a week earlier, they bemoaned having again to laboriously remove every bit of stubble from their bodies. Nonetheless, with the second phase of the ceremony complete, they greatly rejoiced in spirit at their restoration with their families, in spite of their odd appearance. They, indeed, looked remarkably like giant, ruddy, newborn babes when they entered their tents to join their families for the first time since being stricken with the dreaded disease. Indeed, everything seemed new.

After a night spent in the warmth of family, each man made his way to the temple with the animals, grain, and oil that the priest instructed them to bring for the third and final phase of the ceremony of cleansing. Curious onlookers gawked and whispered about the bizarre state of hairless men who made their way through the streets of Jerusalem to the temple. By the time they arrived, the whole city buzzed with the news of ten men whom Jesus had cleansed from leprosy.

[lii] Leviticus 1:9 & 13

Seeing that the men remained blemish free and had complied with all aspects of the washing and shaving, Matthias began to explain the procedures for the final phase of cleansing.

"Men, you have been declared clean and restored to fellowship with your friends and family. However, the most important restoration yet remains, and this final phase will remedy that. I will take the elements that you have provided and offer them on your behalf before the LORD your God."

The priest then took one of the male lambs and slaughtered it according to the Law. "You, what is your name?"

"Joash."

"Joash, my son. Remove your sandal from your right foot. I will now place some of the blood of the guilt offering you have given on the lobe of your right ear, the thumb of your right hand, and the big toe of your right foot. The blood represents forgiveness from sin, and by placing it on these parts of your body, I represent YHWH's sanctification of your entire body. The blood always comes first because without the blood there is no forgiveness of sin."[liii]

The priest silently applied the blood, first on the ear, then on the right thumb, and finally on the right big toe. Oddly enough, the placement of the bright blood now marked a former leper in the same fashion as the priest himself had once been consecrated to the LORD for service.[liv] "Now, I will take some of the oil you have brought and place it in my left hand."

Matthias then sprinkled the oil seven times before the LORD, as the Scriptures directed. Unlike the ceremony that had once ordained him as a priest, Moses' law now specified that Matthias should dip his right forefinger into the oil and place it directly on top of the blood on Joash's ear, hand, and foot.

Afterward, Matthias continued in his explanation, "Finally, with the remaining oil in my palm, I anoint your head."

[liii] Leviticus 17:11 and Hebrews 9:22
[liv] Leviticus 8:23-24

While Joash and the others attempted to control the emotions that flooded their souls, the priest went on to offer, before the LORD, the sin, and burnt offerings, along with the grain offering. When Matthias finished the final requirements of the ceremony of cleansing, he released the men with God's blessing--cleansed, justified, and sanctified. Their joy knew no bounds!

Understanding the Prophetic Tapestry

As I concluded my studies and writing about the ceremony of cleansing from infectious skin diseases, my heart within me wanted to burst forth in a song of praise to my precious, Lord and Savior for all that He has done for you and me! So that you might also be fully blessed by this depth of understanding, I will now further explain the symbolism found within the ceremony.

In individual aspects of the Levitical system, God established partial symbolic pictures that show the need for the atonement for sin and the One who would meet that need. That little-bit-here, little-bit-there approach is a bit like looking through the cracks of a building, which only allows for a partial view from different angles of the marvels inside. But then comes this seemingly unimportant ceremony that was almost never used and that has largely remained in obscurity through the ages. Through that ceremony, it is as though we can throw open the shudders to gain an unobscured view into a room full of wonders.

In the ceremony of cleansing's three phases, God hid an intricately designed picture of the Gospel. As Proverbs 25:2 says, *It is the glory of God to conceal a matter; to search out a matter is the glory of kings.* Today, we can be kings! Join me as I take out my magnifying glass to inspect the individual threads of this tapestry so that we might behold the glory of God.

Each phase focuses on one area where the leper (sinner) needs cleansing so that peace can reign in the entire person. The three areas symbolically portrayed represent the three areas that every individual desperately needs peace to have lasting health. The first phase represents the cleansing of the whole man (spirit, soul, and body), so that man's own heart no longer brings condemnation. This phase pictures the intricate details of salvation through Christ and therefore is the lengthiest of the three phases.

The second phase is brief and merely consists of a repeat of the previous washing and shaving but now in the context of the need for restoration to others. After this second cleansing, the former leper rejoins family and friends in the safe harbor of home. The second cleansing represents an end to the separation between people that occurs because of sin and the fellowship with the family of God that must follow salvation.

Finally, in the third phase Scripture states ten times that the actions taken occur "before the LORD." Such repetition indicates strongly that the cleansed individual requires and now finds right standing before God Almighty. No one can dispute what God has Himself witnessed and established.

Symbols of the Gospel in Phase One

Having now viewed God's prophetic tapestry as a whole, let us direct our focus to the individual threads of the first phase which, when woven together, beautifully picture the Gospel and salvation. Consider the images of Jesus' death in the ritual. Like the first bird in the ceremony, Jesus was crushed and broken (rather than cut like a sacrificial lamb). As represented by the clay bowl into which the bird's blood flows, Jesus' blood was shed for mankind. Even though none of His bones were broken, Jesus spoke of remembering His death through communion in those terms-- *this is my body, which is broken for you.*[iv]

We also see specific pictures of the Messiah's work at the cross through three symbolic elements (cedar wood, hyssop, and scarlet thread). The priest joined them together as one to sprinkle the

---

[iv] 1 Corinthians 11:24 KJV

cleansing blood and water mixture on the former leper. Each of the three symbols has a dual meaning--first to prophesy a detail of the Messiah's unique death and second to represent a spiritual truth.

For instance, the scarlet robe placed on Jesus following a brutal beating where his blood flowed freely found prophetic representation in the scarlet thread.[lvi] That symbol also represents the spiritual cleansing of the blood.[lvii] Similarly, the symbolic hyssop stalk made an appearance in the crucifixion when a soldier offered Jesus a drink from a stalk of hyssop as he hung on the cross.[lviii] Spiritually speaking, the hyssop also represents cleansing from sin.[lix] Likewise, the symbolic wood foretold of the wooden cross on which Jesus died, as well as spiritually representing the curse of God resting on the Messiah in the place of sinful man.[lx] The three symbols foretold of the crucifixion of Jesus and joined as one to picture cleansing for the sinner by the blood and the water.[lxi]

The Blood, the Water, & the Spirit

The unique combination of blood and water in phase one of the ceremony is a distinctive pairing that has great significance in God's prophetic tapestry. They foretold of the literal flow of fluids from Jesus' side when a soldier would one day pierce the Messiah with a spear to confirm His death.[lxii] The apostle John also explains the spiritual significance of the water and the blood in 1 John 5:6. He says, *This is the one who came by water and blood—Jesus Christ. He did not come by water only, but by water and blood.*

[lvi] Matthew 27:28
[lvii] Hebrews 9:22
[lviii] John 19:29
[lix] Psalm 51:7
[lx] Galatians 3:13
[lxi]The priests used these same elements to make the cleansing water for the purification of sin. Numbers 19:1-9
[lxii] John 19:34

However, that verse does not end by simply declaring that Jesus fulfilled the prophecy regarding the water and blood but immediately goes on to point to the Holy Spirit as a witness to the work of Christ. *And it is the Spirit who testifies because the Spirit is the truth.* Understanding the Spirit's role as a witness to the Messiah's work of salvation explains, in part, the symbolic use of birds in the ceremony.

Do you recall the familiar story of John baptizing Jesus, and how the Holy Spirit descended on the Son of God in the form of a bird? Just as the Holy Spirit, seen in that instance as a bird, bore witness to the Son of God, so also the use of birds in the ceremony of cleansing forms a clear image of the Spirit testifying to the sinner's cleansing through Jesus' work at the cross. After all, the living bird provides the means that the priest uses to shake the blood and water seven times onto those made clean.

The 1 John 5 passage goes on to testify to this significance when it says, *The Spirit, the water and the blood; and the three are in agreement* (vs 8). Surely, in writing those words, John had in mind the only Old Testament instance that foreshadowed together the water, blood, and Spirit--the ceremony of cleansing.

The imagery of New Life

I also find the imagery portrayed of resurrection and new life through the Spirit striking. Not only do the two birds, one dead and the other one alive, depict Jesus' death and resurrection but also the believer who was dead in sin and raised to new life. Just picture that scene--the priest releases his death-hold on the bird, who, dazed at first, then shakes off the blood that it might soar freely through the open field. No obstacle blocks its way. Just as Jesus conquered the grave, death binds the sinner no longer!

The birds in the ceremony symbolize the Holy Spirit for another reason as well. The Bible tells us specifically that it is the Spirit of God who accomplishes resurrection and new life. *And if the Spirit of him who raised Jesus from the dead is living in you, he who raised Christ from the dead will also give life to your mortal bodies because of his Spirit who lives in you.*[lxiii] What a fantastic promise that verse makes! The Spirit not only provides new life to the spiritual man but also to the physical man. God could not have portrayed such glorious truth more aptly than He did through the use of the two birds in the ceremony!

Following the imagery of the Gospel in the ceremony, the leper, like the sinner, finds himself/herself declared clean seven times and is reborn. (Seven times is the number of completion in the Bible.) As a final flourish to this phase of the ceremony, God vividly depicts rebirth by requiring that the cleansed leper shave off every hair on his body. I am quite certain that in our modern age of lubricated, four-bladed razors we cannot adequately fathom what God required in this step. Furthermore, to the Jewish man, shaving his beard, say nothing of every hair on his body, would be shameful. However, what better way could there be to give an adult the appearance of a baby when first born into the world?

Consider the words of Jesus to the Pharisee Nicodemus while explaining the need for rebirth through salvation. Notice how closely His explanation mirrors the prophetic picture from the ceremony of cleansing.

> *I tell you the truth, unless a man is born again, he cannot see the kingdom of God. "How can a man be born when he is old?" Nicodemus asked...Jesus answered, "I tell you the truth, unless a man is born of water and the Spirit, he cannot enter the kingdom of God" (John 3:3-5).*

The Oil of Healing

Now, let us jump ahead to consider the significance of the use of oil in the third phase of the ceremony of cleansing. We must not forget that the context of this entire ceremony lies against the backdrop of illness. The Expositor's Bible Commentary states that,

---

[lxiii] Romans 8:11

> *Sickness was symbolic of sin, and even now it should not be
> forgotten that sickness and death are part of God's curse on the
> sin of Adam and his race. Therefore, cleansing the diseased
> person required sacrifices.*[43]

The priest offers four of the five sacrifices from the Levitical law
on behalf of the ceremonially clean individual. During the burnt
offering, the priest must pause to interject a series of bizarre acts--the
placement of blood and oil on the right earlobe, thumb, and big toe.
The placement of the blood in this way occurs elsewhere only in the
ordination ceremony for the priests of God. By using the same
procedure for the cleansed leper following a complete symbolic
portrayal of the Gospel and salvation, we see foreshadowed the
priesthood of believers that Peter speaks of in 1 Peter 2:9.[lxiv] It is
fitting, then, for the cleansed leper (representing a believer) to be
anointed with the blood in the same manner as the priests.

The application of the oil directly on top of the blood, however,
remains unique in all Mosaic Law. (Bear with me now because
understanding the significance of the oil is huge!) In the Old
Testament, the anointing with oil had one use only--to sanctify a person
or object for God's use. Exodus 30:22-33 instructs the priests to make
this oil from a secret recipe of spices mixed with oil. Any who tried to
use this oil for personal use were to be cut off from God's people. Plain
olive oil, on the other hand, represented God's blessing and had many
uses, including being a component of offerings.

The meaning and use of anointing oil, however, expanded with
Jesus. Psalm 45:7 speaks of the Father anointing the Son of God with
the oil of gladness or joy. Hebrews 1:9 tells us that Jesus fulfilled that
passage. The prophet Isaiah also prophesied of the Father anointing

---

[lxiv] *But you are a chosen people, a royal priesthood, a holy nation, God's
special possession, that you may declare the praises of him who called you out
of darkness into his wonderful light.*

His Son but then goes on to speak of the Son bestowing on others that same oil of gladness.[lxv]

From the beginning, God intended that Jesus would usher in a change--*the year of the LORD's favor*.[lxvi] Jesus claimed to be the fulfillment of that prophecy from Isaiah before all of those in attendance for worship at a synagogue in Nazareth.[lxvii] Not long afterward, without any explanation, Jesus' disciples suddenly used oil to anoint sick people for purposes of healing while on their first missionary journey.[lxviii] The oil used would not have been the official anointing oil but instead olive oil, just as was used in the ceremony of cleansing.[lxix] Anointing people with oil for healing had never been seen in Scripture before. Why the change?

The Blood and the Oil

The ceremony of cleansing gives us the answer in a prophetic picture. Through the application of the blood and the oil, following a clear portrayal of salvation, we see the means of healing that God intended to institute following Christ's work at the cross. In light of the powerful imagery of the bird taking flight in the ceremony of cleansing, consider the very last passage of the Old Testament as spoken by the prophet Malachi regarding the coming Messiah. *But for you who revere my name, the sun of righteousness will rise with healing in its rays. And you will go out and frolic like well-fed calves.*[lxx]

The prophet says this benefit of healing through Jesus would be for those who revere His name (believers). Just as David praises God for the benefits of both the forgiveness of sin and the healing of disease

---

[lxv] Isaiah 61:3
[lxvi] Isaiah 61:2 and Luke 4:19
[lxvii] Luke 4:16-21
[lxviii] Mark 6:13
[lxix] We know this because Exodus 30:33 commands that no person, other than a priest be anointed with the Levitical anointing oil.
[lxx] Malachi 4:2

in Psalm 103:3, so also, we see that healing would be an ongoing benefit for believers, tied directly to sanctification--hence the oil is applied directly on top of the blood in the ceremony. Dear brother or sister, we must not forget this principle: **Since the time of Christ, sanctification and healing have gone together**. (I will discuss many passages in future chapters that emphasize this truth first pictured in the ceremony of cleansing.)

C. I. Scofield, an American theologian, suggests that oil in the Bible represents the Holy Spirit. A case for this can be made when we consider that the year of the Lord's favor ushered in the gift of the Holy Spirit that would indwell all believers. Certainly, the oil, which undoubtedly represents the anointing with God's blessing could also represent the anointing by the Spirit. As we saw in Romans 8:11, the same Spirit who breathed life into Jesus for resurrection also breathes life into our mortal bodies. Therefore, anointing the sick person with oil is representative of God's blessing of healing through the Holy Spirit's life-giving power.

In James 5:14-16, God instructs sick believers to go to the elders, who should then anoint them with oil and pray for them. I must emphasize again though, that the blood for forgiveness must precede the oil of healing, which is why verses fifteen and sixteen speak of confession and forgiveness in conjunction with healing.

Is anyone among you sick? Let them call the elders of the church to pray over them and anoint them with oil in the name of the Lord. And the prayer offered in faith will make the sick person well; the Lord will raise them up. If they have sinned, they will be forgiven. Therefore, confess your sins to each other and pray for each other so that you may be healed. The prayer of a righteous person is powerful and effective.

The question arises, then, whether or not one must be anointed with oil to be healed? No. Jesus and the apostles healed many people without anointing them with oil. However, God did not, without reason, instruct us through James to seek the elders for this purpose.

Therefore, obedience is wise. I took this step of faith when I was sick, but unfortunately, the elders did not attempt to discuss the need for confession and repentance that James spoke of in conjunction with the anointing of oil and prayer. It would be another year before God brought to my attention my need for repentance, at which time He healed me. Never forget: The believer's benefit of healing follows the application of the blood of forgiveness.

Our Future Hope

To complete the showcasing of God's prophetic tapestry, I must mention one remaining thread--that of the one missing sacrifice. Of the five types of offerings, only the peace (or fellowship) offering remains absent from the ceremony of cleansing. This voluntary offering would typically follow the others and represents the eating of a meal between the LORD and the individual.[lxxi] Perhaps, the intentional absence of the peace offering from the ceremony of cleansing was to picture prophetically the future hope for all whom God cleanses. Revelation 19:9 exclaims, *Blessed are those who are invited to the wedding supper of the Lamb!"*

Voila! All of the threads of different colors and textures, which seem meaningless on their own, weave together to form God's prophetic masterpiece revealing the work of Christ at the cross--the forgiveness of sin and the healing of disease. The apostle Paul beautifully summarizes that work on our behalf in 1 Corinthians 6:11. *And that is what some of you were. But you were washed, you were sanctified, you were justified in the name of the Lord Jesus Christ and by the Spirit of our God.* Praise be to God!

[lxxi] Leviticus 7:11-21

Biblical Principle: *Since the time of Christ, sanctification and healing have gone together.*

Call to Action: *Take some time to worship the Lord with a thankful heart for all that He has accomplished for you.*

CHAPTER 9

Peace With God

Whoever is wise, let him heed these things and consider the great love of the Lord. Psalm 107:43

A new day dawns and the familiar routine begins in assisting my husband with getting out the door for another day of work. With a kiss, he is off, and then I am free to privately indulge my longing to spend time over a cup of coffee with the other Love of my life.

Nestled into my comfy recliner with a view of birds and flowers out my window, I settle in to spend time with the lover of my soul. This is the time for which I live. I am always amazed, as I listen and consider His thoughts, how brilliant and insightful He is, and I wonder why the Lord of the universe would bother to share His thoughts with the likes of me.

Sometimes I am distracted, I admit, but He patiently waits while I determine to set aside other preoccupations and hear what He has for me. When He shares something that moves me, He never seems uncomfortable with my emotions. Furthermore, if I find something He says confusing, He always responds with patient clarification when I ask for it. Clearly, He longs for this private time with me as well, although I will never understand why.

Not wanting to end my time with the One I love but needing a change in venue, I exchange my empty coffee cup for a pair of athletic shoes, and we set off together on a walk or run. Mile after mile we traverse the neighborhoods surrounding my house, enjoying the morning and lost in private conversation. He listens to me talk about whatever is on my mind, and I try to remember not to be so much of a chatterbox that He does not have a chance to respond with His insights. Every moment in His presence fills me with joy! *My lover is mine, and I am his* (Song of Songs 2:16). What a wonderful thing that is!

It was not always this way. In fact, it was only in recent years that I became aware that He truly loved me. Imagine One so fine choosing me! I thought that He would only send a smile my way if I diligently worked for Him, so I tried endlessly to serve Him. In spite of significant health struggles, day after day and year after year, I slaved for Him, hoping to earn His pleasure. I became His champion, but privately my resentment that He seemed so relentless in His demands interfered with tender moments. "Why can He not just love me for myself and not for all I do for Him?" I wondered. It must be because of my countless flaws and failures, I reasoned. So, I determined to try harder.

However, life became increasingly more difficult. New trials appeared around every corner in endless succession. From my limited perspective, it seemed that He met all of my efforts to please Him with judgment. Why could He love others but not me? Was I really so awful? All of these thoughts drove a wedge deeper between us, separating me further from the love I craved. Day after day, I contemplated why God had it out for me.

Finally, I shared my struggle with a Christian counselor. Surprisingly, she recognized the heart of the matter immediately. She pointed out that I had a huge volume of love letters from Him, which spoke of His unfailing and unconditional love for me, but I was choosing not to believe them. I had been behaving as though I could earn His love, and so His only recourse was to take me to a place where I literally could not DO anything except to draw near and listen. She wisely challenged me to keep reading those love letters but to look for any tender words of affection and make the conscious choice to believe every word. So, I did.

She was right! His letters (the Bible) were full of declarations of His undying love for me! Slowly, His words began to seep into my consciousness and renew me. How could I have missed it all those years? I wanted to shout it from the rooftops. I am loved! I am loved because my Lover chose me, just for me, and not because of something I could do for Him! He thinks I am beautiful! He has forgiven me for all of my failings and wants me to know Him as no one else knows Him.

Oh, to be loved! It changes a person. She who is loved much is now free to love much in return. My lover is mine, and I am his.

My First Round of Healing

In the months following the counselor's challenge, God's Word and Spirit radically transformed my heart from one that desperately feared the future due to my view of a wrathful God, to a heart that swam in the deep waters of God's limitless love. Despite the continued problems with pain and illness, joy began to fill my days. The sound of melodious hymns flowed from my lips as I worked around the house, and changes in my health surfaced. How true it is that *a heart at peace gives life to the body*.[lxxii] By removing the tremendous and previously unending stress response due to the feeling that God was against me, my body began to be rejuvenated.

As is so often the case when God works mightily, the enemy doubles his efforts to undermine that work. Such was the case with me in this next phase of my journey. It shames me to admit how I fell prey to Satan's deception, but I choose to share anyway because I know the desperation of those who suffer from poor health, and the tremendous temptation alleged solutions present.

[lxxii] Proverbs 14:30

Ironically, following the time of great healing in my relationship with the Lord, I became unknowingly involved with demonic practices. It would be almost two years before my eyes would be opened to see behind the veil, so to speak. My journey into Satan's deception began with a visit to the local library. I noticed a book on display that grabbed my attention with a title that promised health. It spoke of something I had never heard of before involving a practice of testing and treating allergies using muscle testing, or Applied Kinesiology (AK).[lxxiii] It theorized that all illness resulted from allergies. The book claimed that by using these practices, one could forever be cured of any allergies, and therefore, any symptom or illness. Intrigued, I sought out a practitioner in my area and went for my first appointment.

Although the whole thing sounded a bit crazy and the appointment was strange, I was desperate for physical solutions. Shockingly, the initial results were dramatic, even miraculous. My first treatment made me feel like I had the flu for a couple of days, but I was used to strong, negative reactions to everything I tried, so I determined to go again anyway. The next treatment for calcium seemed to make a significant difference in my sleep. Even though I had serious misgivings about the nature of the testing and treatments, I went back a third time.

This time, following treatment for iodine, my thyroid immediately began to function normally. I kid you not! I had been on thyroid medication for nearly three years at this point but had to stop taking it immediately because my normal thyroid function returned. Normalcy plus medication equaled hyperthyroidism, which produced a terribly racing heart.

According to conventional medical understanding, once an individual is on thyroid medication, that person can never get off of it

---

[lxxiii] Applied Kinesiology is one of many forms of a large number of alternative medical practices now labeled as energetic medicine. I will explain and discuss at length in chapter 17--*Spiritual Forces and Health,* why I am certain these practices make use of demonic forces. Even though my story will likely raise many questions, in this chapter my only focus will be on how AK played into my health story. See Appendix E for an explanation of AK.

because the natural function of the thyroid largely ceases as it relies almost solely on the medication. However, for the first time in many years, including while being on the medication, I had normal thyroid function, which remains to this day.

You can imagine my shock! Even though an undeniable sense of unease over the practice of muscle testing and related treatments pervaded my thoughts, I wrongly concluded that AK must be of God. After all, I reasoned--He appeared to have used it to heal my thyroid, and *every good and perfect gift is from above*.[lxxiv] I failed to consider that a merciful and sovereign God might orchestrate my healing because of changes in my heart towards Himself, IN SPITE OF my ignorant decision to get involved with AK. Such grace in no way legitimizes the practices I became involved with, but instead testifies to a loving Father who had mercy on His child as she fumbled in the dark. (I will offer a more thorough analysis of the "healing" of my thyroid and the consequences of my involvement with AK in chapter seventeen.)

Because the AK treatments for everything other than my thyroid regularly failed, I needed to repeat previous treatments continuously. I learned to do it all myself and taught my family members as well so that I could manage my symptoms at home. I became quite proficient in AK as a result and additionally began treating others.

Separately, but also during this time, I learned information on back stretches and exercises that quickly proved effective in reducing the inflammation and pain associated with my injured spine. Additionally, I discovered in the days, months, and years ahead that all of my female related conditions disappeared, including a fibroid and endometriosis. For the first time in my life, my monthly cycles brought only the mildest cramps. My body's hormone production had come into balance.

Although I had some other physical conditions that remained, for the first time in seventeen years, I could function near normalcy. After

---

[lxxiv] James 1:17

a year of barely being able to stand long enough to brush my teeth, I was soon running miles at a time in the heat of summer. Less than a year later, I taught third-grade full time and kept a rigorous schedule. I could never have dreamed that God would bring such changes to pass. However, it would be almost two years before I would come to understand the connection between the heartfelt knowledge of the Lord's love for me and the physical healing that occurred.

To Thrive Everyone Needs Love

The Creator of the universe fashioned our inmost being to need love desperately. After all, the God of love did make us in His image! That intrinsic need for love manifests itself from day one. As a result of multiple studies, modern medicine links *failure to thrive*, which describes an infant who fails to gain weight and develop normally, to a lack of affection.   Scientists--who do not wish to acknowledge a creator--find the human need for love a mystery, and yet many case studies, both intentional and accidental, have repeatedly established that humans require love to thrive.

An Italian Franciscan monk by the name of Salimbene recorded one particularly noteworthy and tragic "study" of infants that occurred in his time by Frederick II of Hohenstaufen. This not-so-holy Roman emperor of the 1200s held many titles and much power. Although excommunicated twice by the papacy, this emperor and king of Germany, Sicily, and Jerusalem held an endless fascination with living things. Lacking a moral code and having no one to stand in his way, Frederick's pursuit of an empirical understanding of biology provided the catalyst to macabre experiments, which a disapproving Salimbene recorded in The Twelve Calamities Of Emperor Frederick II. The most notorious of these studies involved infants.

Being convinced of the supremacy of Germans, Frederick believed the German language must have been originally spoken in the Garden of Eden and determined to prove his theory. Understanding nothing about language acquisition, Frederick reasoned that if an infant were not predisposed to any particular language, he would then begin spontaneously to utter the original language of Adam and Eve.

According to the monk, the emperor gave strict orders on how to care for a group of infants to some nurses. Not a word or a cooing might be uttered by the ladies, and only the most minimal of contact might be given through feeding and bathing the unfortunate souls. The king would never attain his answer about language because the infants reportedly died from starvation, not from lack of food but love. Although no empirical record exists of the numbers of children involved or other specific details, save the testimony of Salimbene, other historical records lend credence to the monk's reports.[44]

In more modern times, a pediatrician by the name of Dr. Harry Bakwin recorded his observations of the children in New York's Bellevue Hospital in 1942. The hospital had an alarmingly high mortality rate, which was attributed to malnutrition and infection. In an attempt to prevent the spread of bacteria to its smallest patients, children were placed in small cubicles and attended to by completely covered nurses and physicians who were instructed, *to move about cautiously so as to not stir up bacteria.*[45] The mortality rate persisted, and in spite of the high-caloric intake of the children, they failed to gain weight until returning home. Finally, the hospital changed its policies and encouraged nurses to love-on the kids and allowed parents to visit. In spite of the potential for germ exposure, the children's mortality rate dropped from 30-35% to less than 10%.[46]

Examples that demonstrate the fundamental human need for love and the catastrophic physical impact when it is lacking abound. From the cradle to the grave, nothing robs us of peace, and therefore, health, like a pervading sense that we are not loved! Most accept that this proves true in human relationships, but I would contend that it proves equally true in our relationship with God.

The Innate Need for God's Love

St. Augustine of Hippo emphasized the fundamental need for peace with God in a quote for which he is famous: *You have formed us for Yourself, and our hearts are restless till they find rest in You.*[47] The Bible speaks of how God placed this need for Him in us so that our restlessness might lead us to a right relationship with him. ***God did this so that they would seek him and perhaps reach out for him and find him, though he is not far from any one of us. 'For in him we live and move and have our being'*** (Acts 17:27-28).

If everyone has an innate need for God's love, what happens to that need when, upon salvation, one becomes a child of God? Surely, the desire for His love must then increase significantly. After all, God created us FOR Himself, and with salvation, He becomes our Father, Friend, and Savior. Just as one feels the need for love greater in a close, earthly relationship than in a casual one, so also does one sense the need for God's love and approval increasingly more following salvation. When the Christian rests secure in the Father's love, peace and joy fill the heart to overflowing.

However, the certainty of that love can diminish over time when the hardness of life, Satan's lies, bad doctrine, or numerous other things manage to call into question the Father's love and create false views of Him. Such trials can even undermine our foundation of faith and erode the heart's sense of peace. Do any of the following false views of God resonate with you?

- He expects me to be perfect and is just waiting for me to mess up so He can punish me.

- He remains distant and does not care what happens to me.

- He only loves those who are "good" Christians.

- It does not matter what I do because He will forgive my sin.

- He is angry with me.

The Physical Impact of God's Love

I introduced Psalm 16:8-11 in chapter one but only in the general context of the "path of life." Let us now look again at those verses and get more specific.

> *I keep my eyes always on the Lord. With him at my right hand, I will not be shaken. Therefore, my heart is glad, and my tongue rejoices; my body also will rest secure, because you will not abandon me to the realm of the dead, nor will you let your faithful one see decay. You make known to me the path of life; you will fill me with joy in your presence, with eternal pleasures at your right hand.*

These verses speak of walking the path of life, near the Lord, eyes focused on Him, and with Him at the right hand (metaphorically indicating His position of strength). Consider that type of walk for a moment. Would you willingly walk close to someone you mistrust? Certainly not! What about someone you believe has rejected you or who is mean, angry, or cruel? The close walk depicted in these verses portrays a deep trust and love between the two parties.

According to this passage, some wonderful things become true of the individual who enjoys a close walk with the loving Savior, namely joy, peace, a glad heart, a rejoicing tongue, and a secure body. Such desirable blessings come to pass when fear and doubt disappear and peace reigns. With fear absent, joy alone remains in the presence of the Father. Therefore, this Psalm beautifully highlights the next Biblical principle of health: **Resting in God's love brings joy and health.**

As I once did, many people struggle with a wide assortment of wrong views about God's character. Just this past week, I spoke at length with two women who wrestle in the depths of their being with the belief that God has rejected them. From what I could discern, both have truly placed their faith in Christ alone for salvation, and both have a tremendous knowledge of Scripture. And yet, both agonize over the certainty that they have sinned too much for God to forgive.

It is not that either has sinned worse than your average individual, but that their childhoods, bad Bible teaching, and the significant hardships of their life experiences cloud their ability to rest in their heavenly Father. Fear of God's judgment and wrath color every promise and assurance of His love for them. Therefore, God's Word seems more like a club than a soothing ointment. It was no surprise then to learn that both suffer tremendously from significant physical conditions. My heart broke for these women whom the devil torments with lies.

As I explained in chapters four and five, the physical heart responds profoundly to a lack of peace, sending out messages that negatively impact the autonomic nervous system and thereby the entire body. God created us to be in close fellowship with Him, so our hearts, which need peace, alert us physically when something interferes with that fellowship so that we might return to His loving arms.

Sin can, of course, prevent fellowship, but so also can wrong views of God's character. I had no idea when I first went to the Christian counselor that my view of God had any connection to my physical pain and suffering. Furthermore, I never dreamed that once God's Word transformed my wrong thinking about the Father, God would heal my physical body of all of my hormone-related conditions. However, that is what He did.

God wired women as particularly emotional beings. We feel things greatly. During the time of Jesus' ministry, it was women who threw caution to the wind and loved Jesus with abandon. Just consider how Mary poured out a perfume that cost a year's wages to anoint Jesus' feet. It was the women, whose love superseded thoughts of self-preservation, who were present at the crucifixion. Unlike the women, the male disciples, save John, feared too much for their safety to stand watch until the end. The women were also first at Jesus' tomb. It is this beautiful abandon in a woman's heart that also leaves her the most vulnerable to illness when she does not feel loved.

As discussed in chapter five, hormones are the autonomic nervous system's first responders to thoughts and emotions. It seems reasonable then to generalize that a woman's hormones are more greatly affected than men's from feeling unloved. (This holds true when women lack a sense of love from any key relationship, whether it be their father, husband, or God.) That is not to say that men do not also need love, but only that, because of God's design, women sense the need more acutely. Therefore, it makes sense that the female hormones, key to femininity, would be the primary target for imbalance when a woman does not experience love.

Loving God Takes First Priority

If you recall, the three phases of the ceremony of cleansing from infectious disease portray the need for cleansing within oneself, with others, and with God. In Mark 12:29-31, Jesus prioritized those three relationships by stating that loving God comes first.

> *Hear, O Israel: The Lord our God, the Lord is one. Love the Lord your God with all your heart and with all your soul and with all your mind and with all your strength. The second is this: 'Love your neighbor as yourself.*

Did you notice in the opening statement we are reminded of the unified nature of God (the Lord is one)? Just as the Godhead stands unified, so also God desires unity in each of the three relationships where man is commanded to demonstrate love. First and foremost, He commands us to love Him with our entire being (heart, soul, mind, and strength).[lxxv] How can every aspect of our person be united in a love of the Father when an accurate understanding of His character is missing? The apostle Paul spoke of the connection between knowing God and loving Him in a prayer found in a letter to the Philippian church. He said, *And this is my prayer: that your love may abound more and more in knowledge and depth of insight.*[lxxvi] The more we know God, the more we love Him. Knowledge must be based on truth.

[lxxv] We shall cover the 2nd command in later chapters.
[lxxvi] Philippians 1:9

Correcting False Views of God

Peoples' hearts filter truth according to personal experiences and emotions, and the unwanted result is often that the truth of God's love is not grasped. Coming to an awareness of one's personal biases can open the way for the truth to permeate the walls of the heart and bring healing. So, what skews your ability to rest in the love of the Father?

Often the cause of false views of God comes from an earthly father who badly represented the role of fatherhood to his children. Of all the things to which God could compare Himself, it seems odd that He would have chosen the role of fatherhood. Just think about the biblical fathers. They were all lousy! And yet, throughout time God places imperfect men into the weighty role of reflecting a heavenly Father who loves unconditionally, unfailingly, patiently, mercifully, and who continually demonstrates grace to His children.

Very few individuals have the privilege of being raised by a father who even slightly reflects the traits of God the Father. Recognition of where one has transposed their earthly father's faulty character onto the Lord is a good starting place for healing. Then, it is imperative that the truth of God's love, found in His Word, rewrite the negative patterns of thought.

A second major area that frequently produces false views of God comes from the pain and suffering that life so often brings. Because trials have a cumulative effect, each new tragedy in life can bring one increasingly into struggle with his/her Maker. Rather than being thought of as isolated incidents, each new hardship compounds the pain of previous struggles. In this way, over time, the addition of minor hardships, say nothing of major ones, seems monumental and adds "evidence" that God cannot be trusted as loving and good.

As a result, even in good times, one feels they are holding their breath, just waiting for something to go wrong. Since the Bible teaches of God's sovereignty, it can be easy to determine that God must be cruel, angry, and certainly not good since He has allowed such personal suffering. Trust flies out the window! This lack of peace with God produces great fear and tremendously impacts one's physical health.

Regardless of their origin, the answer to false views of God lies in knowing Him in truth. Keep in mind that many inaccurate views of God have their basis in truth. For example, we know according to Scripture that God is holy, our judge, and full of wrath. However, is that the entire picture? For someone who had a cruel father or a hard life, the attributes related to God's holiness can easily take prominence rather than being seen in the light of God's love and goodness. As a result, the truth of God's nature is lost to the heart.

Upon recognizing such a bias, one can replace their improper perspective of God's judgment with the knowledge that the heavenly Father met the need for justice for our sin with the blood of His own Son. By so doing, He proved His unconditional love. Therefore, anyone who has placed their trust in Jesus' payment for sin no longer faces condemnation, judgment, or wrath.[lxxvii] This is only one example of how to take into account God's total character, rather than allowing one facet to outweigh another, thereby altering the truth.

The misrepresentation of who God is has a long history. In fact, Satan has never been opposed to twisting God's Word to portray the Lord falsely. ***Did God really say...*** Genesis 3:1. Also consider the story of Satan tempting Jesus after He had fasted in the wilderness for forty days.[lxxviii] The devil employed Scripture, taken out of context or in exclusion of other Scriptures, to try and mislead the Savior.

What was Jesus' response to Satan's deceptive use of God's Word? Was it not to quote back a different passage that put in place the proper context of the first passage? Satan often uses the same tactic to mislead those who know Scripture, and we must respond as Jesus did. The next section lists correct views of God's character along with one example from Scripture to support each view. (Appendix B contains an expanded list of verses to help further.)

[lxxvii] Romans 8:1
[lxxviii] Matthew 4:1-10

God loves me personally.

- Psalm 66:20, *Praise be to God, who has not rejected my prayer or withheld his love from me!*

God's love is NOT based on my performance.

- Psalm 103:13-15 & 17, *...the LORD has compassion on those who fear him, for he knows how we are formed, he remembers that we are dust. As for man, his days are like grass...But from everlasting the LORD's love is with those who fear him.*

If my faith is in Christ, God is NOT waiting to judge and condemn me.

- Romans 8:1-2, *Therefore, there is now no condemnation for those who are in Christ Jesus, because through Christ Jesus the law of the Spirit who gives life has set you free from the law of sin and death.*

God sees my suffering, cares, and will work on my behalf.

- Isaiah 51:3, *The Lord will surely comfort Zion and will look with compassion on all her ruins; he will make her deserts like Eden, her wastelands like the garden of the Lord. Joy and gladness will be found in her, thanksgiving and the sound of singing.*

If I have failed to address the particular false view of God that you struggle with, just follow my example, and find Scriptures that counter this false view or add the appropriate context.

Never forget that this is a spiritual battle for your heart, which greatly impacts your health, and so it should not be ignored. Paul's words in 2 Corinthians 10:3-5 remind us of the steps to transforming the mind described in chapter seven.[lxxix]

[lxxix] Easily reference the steps in Appendix 3.

For though we live in the world, we do not wage war as the world does. The weapons we fight with are not the weapons of the world. On the contrary, they have divine power to demolish strongholds. We demolish arguments and every pretension that sets itself up against the knowledge of God, and we take captive every thought to make it obedient to Christ.

Although following the Apostle's instructions for transforming the mind might seem difficult, take encouragement from how quickly neuroplastic change can come about when the brain is not allowed to continue down the old ruts.

If you struggle with trusting God's love for you, I strongly encourage you to set this book aside for a while to read my book, When You Can't Trust His Heart--Discovering the Limitless Love of God and simultaneously work through the corresponding study guide. I cannot emphasize enough the importance of dealing fully with this issue because resting in God's love brings joy and health. Determine today to address the most important relationship in your life. Then you, too, will find your tongue rejoicing and your spirit longing for the presence of God while your body rests secure.

My lover is mine, and I am his. Oh, the joy such knowledge brings!

Biblical Principle: *Resting in God's love brings joy and health.*

Call to Action: *Consider whether you have any skewed or wrong views of God that prevent you from trusting Him fully. If you do, use the verses in Appendix B, combined with the three steps for transforming the mind found in Appendix C, to align your thinking with the biblical portrayal of God's character and His love for you.*

CHAPTER 10

Sanctification & Health

Therefore, this is what the Lord Almighty says: "See, I will refine and test them, for what else can I do because of the sin of my people?" Jeremiah 9:7

After God healed me of all my hormone-related conditions and back pain, I could live again. That statement might sound cliché unless you know first-hand the severely diminished quality of life that comes with poor health, causing the desire "to live again" to fill every waking longing. Without fibromyalgia, hypothyroidism, a spine in pain, and monthly cycles ruling and severely limiting my options, God opened many doors to me that once seemed dead-bolted shut. I also had a closeness with my Savior brought to pass by a deep awareness of His unfailing and boundless love for me.

However, one significant problem area remained--I now seemed to be allergic to everything. These "allergies" caused numerous daily interruptions because I physically reacted in a variety of ways to almost everything I ate, breathed, and touched. The reactions were short-lived though, due to my proficiency in testing and treating using Applied Kinesiology (AK). I imagine God cringed every time I thanked Him for this "gift" that allowed me only fleeting relief from reactions because He knew the true nature of the constant bondage Satan had brought me into, and the lasting deliverance God alone could bring.

About a year and a half into that two-year period, the Lord brought a new friendship into my life. We were quite different in age and personality but kindred spirits in our love for the Father, and much of our conversation centered around Him. A wonderful quirk of hers included a passion for books but not in the typical sense. She preferred to read the last chapter first to see if it caught her interest and then read random sections but never the whole thing. If the book struck her as worthwhile, she then loved to buy multiple copies and give them to anyone she thought could benefit from the content. In this way, she gave me two books that had a profound impact on my life.

The first one she "gifted" me centered around a belief that the Bible teaches that most illnesses have a spiritual root to them. As I mentioned in chapter one, this lengthy book offended me at the outset. "How dare my friend insinuate that my past illnesses and my current issues with allergies might be the result of sin in my life!" She tried to gracefully point out that even though AK allowed me to continue living "normally," it consumed my attention and kept me a slave to it. I heartily disagreed and set the volume on a shelf, determined not to give it another thought.

However, with the loving Lord at work in me, I was unable to rid my mind of the thought that my allergies might have a spiritual component. So early one Saturday morning, while my family slept in, I began to read the book. Although I have now come to different conclusions than the author on some of the content, at the time God used the abundant Scriptures quoted in the book to grab my attention. That morning of reading precipitated a time, as I described in chapter one, of great searching for understanding in the pages of the Bible as to whether or not most illnesses have a spiritual root. I became obsessed with the topic and spent countless hours a day reading.

As I read through the Bible, highlighting in blue every verse that spoke of health, illness, or healing, I came to the book of Jeremiah. A number of the Lord's messages to the Israelites through Jeremiah spoke of God using illness as a means of bringing His people to repentance. Rather than those passages coming across as diatribes, they reveal a deep sorrow on the Lord's part in having to use illness as a tool for restoring His people to Himself. God's heart of grief and longing fill the pages. Furthermore, His warnings often end by expressing a desire to heal them, if they would only repent.

While reading one morning, I came across a detailed private conversation between Jeremiah and God that spoke directly to me. The passage spoke of the prophet's insistence that he lived righteously and therefore should not be suffering physical pain and illness. The fact that Jeremiah was sick surprised me. His complaint about his condition dripped with pride for his righteous living, and I related. Surely, I too could make a similar case to God. Look what the prophet said in 15:15-17:

> *Lord, you understand; remember me and care for me...think of how I suffer reproach for your sake. When your words came, I ate them; they were my joy and my heart's delight, for I bear your name, Lord God Almighty. I never sat in the company of revelers, never made merry with them; I sat alone because your hand was on me and you had filled me with indignation.*

Immediately following Jeremiah's self-righteous reminders to God, he asked the question in verse eighteen that I too had wondered in light of my self-assessment: *Why is my pain unending and my wound grievous and incurable? You are to me like a deceptive brook, like a spring that fails.* "Yes!" I resounded. "I have tried to honor you, Lord, in everything. Surely you have wrongly struck me down all of these years."

But then I read God's response to Jeremiah in verse nineteen. Because the prophet's argument so closely depicted my thinking at the time, it was as if I, not Jeremiah, had spoken the protest and God now answered me directly. *Therefore this is what the Lord says: "If you repent, I will restore you that you may serve me."* Yikes! Because I had always attempted to do what would please the Lord, I had grown proud and self-righteous, just like the prophet. Just as he wrongly compared himself to the rebellious Israelites and became puffed up, so too had I compared myself to the sinful world around me and became noxious in my self-righteousness, critical spirit, and judgment of others.

Oh, how blind I had been to the significance of my sin and the need for the Lord to use illness to bring me to repentance. There in the privacy of my room that morning, I wept over my pride and sought my Savior's forgiveness.

Once the Lord opened my eyes to recognize some of my sin, I became more interested in the multitude of passages connecting sin and illness. As I mentioned, many of those verses also go on to promise God's healing following repentance (more detail on that in the next chapter). When I say that there is a multitude of passages that link sin to illness, I do not exaggerate. In fact, of all the biblical passages on illness and healing, the vast majority make this connection.

In fact, their sheer quantity, great length, and directness can be overwhelming and calls to question why pastors and Bible teachers fail to address this issue. The primary reason, of course, is simple. These passages are offensive. We live in a culture that screams, "Tolerance!" at all times and which loudly condemns calling anything sin. To suggest that parishioners may be sick and dying because of a pattern of sin in their lives might empty the pews. Furthermore, Scripture does give two incontrovertible examples of illnesses that were not the result of sin. In light of those exceptions, a blanket teaching that suggests all who are sick find themselves in that situation because of sin could prove inaccurate and hurtful to those who already suffer greatly. (I will cover these exceptions in chapter sixteen.)

However, teachers of the Bible do have a responsibility before God to teach the Word so that His people will not perish. So out of a heavy burden that I carry for the physical suffering of God's children and a humble heart of love, allow me to share with you some of the passages from the Bible on sin and illness. Please do not see this teaching as condemnation or a lack of empathy for your pain. Instead, it comes from a strong desire that others might also be healed from illnesses resulting from a lack of peace with God due to sin.

Teaching on Illness Due To Sin

Because so many biblical passages emphatically state a connection between sin and illness, I will simply list a few of the many possible passages and let the Word of God speak for itself. Keep in mind that I do not do this to wield God's Word as a club. Just as a surgeon's scalpel must cause pain to bring healing, so also the Bible must at times divide between soul and spirit to bring wholeness. I ask that you bear with me as I quote some lengthy sections of the Bible in this chapter. It just so happens that the passages on this topic tend to be long and to cut them short would sacrifice their weight. I have also underlined specific parts of the body, as well as any ailments mentioned. I do so in order that you might notice the wide-spread, physical impact of sin that the biblical authors describe.

- Psalm 38:1-10 & 17-18 *Lord, do not rebuke me in your anger or discipline me in your wrath. Your arrows have pierced me, and your hand has come down on me. Because of your wrath, there is no health in my body; there is <u>no soundness in my bones</u> because of my sin. My guilt has overwhelmed me like a burden too heavy to bear. My <u>wounds fester</u> and are loathsome because of my sinful folly. I am bowed down and brought very low; all day long I go about mourning. My <u>back is filled with searing pain</u>; there is <u>no health</u> in my body. I am <u>feeble</u> and utterly crushed; I groan in anguish of <u>heart</u>. All my longings lie open before you, Lord; my sighing is not hidden from you. <u>My heart pounds</u>, my <u>strength fails</u> me; even the <u>light has gone from my eyes</u>. For I am about to fall, and my <u>pain is ever with me</u>. I confess my iniquity; I am troubled by my sin.*

- Psalm 32:1-5 *Blessed is the one whose transgressions are forgiven, whose sins are covered. Blessed is the one whose sin* *the Lord does not count against them and in whose spirit is no deceit. When I kept silent, my <u>bones wasted away</u> through my groaning all day long. For day and night your hand was heavy on me, my <u>strength was sapped</u> as in the heat of summer. Then I acknowledged my sin to you and did not cover up my iniquity. I said, "I will confess my transgressions to the Lord." And you forgave the guilt of my sin.*

• Isaiah 1:4-6 *They have forsaken the Lord; they have spurned the Holy One of Israel and turned their backs on him. Why should you be beaten anymore? Why do you persist in rebellion? Your whole <u>head</u> is injured, your whole <u>heart</u> afflicted. From the sole of your <u>foot</u> to the top of your <u>head</u> there is no soundness—only <u>wounds</u> and <u>welts</u> and <u>open sores</u>, not cleansed or bandaged or soothed with olive oil.*

• Jeremiah 9:7 *Therefore, this is what the Lord Almighty says: "See, I will refine and test them, for what else can I do because of the sin of my people?"*

Many more similarly descriptive Old Testament passages could be listed, but you get the idea. At first, when I encountered such verses, I assumed the physical symptoms mentioned were merely figurative expressions. However, while rapidly reading and highlighting the Bible, the frequency of such references, even in non-poetic passages, changed that initial assumption.

Do Those Old Testament Teachings Still Apply?

It is funny how much effort we will expend to try to explain away things we do not want to accept as true. Such was the case with me regarding the connection between sin and illness. So, my attempts to explain it away continued, but this time I focused on the possibility that the connection only held true under the old covenant of the law. If so, now that we are no longer under the law but under grace, we would not need to be concerned with the possibility that God still uses illness as a means of sanctification.[lxxx]

The covenant of the law, to which I refer, was given through Moses in the book of Deuteronomy. Before the Israelites entered the Promised Land, God spelled out the blessings and curses of the covenant. God made it quite simple. If His people obeyed the law of God, then He would bless them in every way imaginable. However, if they rebelled against the Lord and His commands, He would punish them in every conceivable way, including with every form of illness. This listing of specific afflictions is literal and shows the degree and wide assortment of ways that God can impact the normal, physical processes of the human body. Even though it is lengthy, I encourage you to read it afresh.

However, if you do not obey the Lord your God and do not carefully follow all his commands and decrees I am giving you today, all these curses will come on you and overtake you: The Lord will plague you with diseases until he has destroyed you from the land you are entering to possess. The Lord will strike you with wasting disease, with fever and inflammation...until you perish.

The Lord will afflict you with the boils of Egypt and with tumors, festering sores, and the itch, from which you cannot be cured. The Lord will afflict you with madness, blindness, and confusion of mind...The Lord will afflict your knees and legs with painful boils that cannot be cured, spreading from the soles of your feet to the top of your head.

If you do not carefully follow all the words of this law, which are written in this book, and do not revere this glorious and awesome name—the Lord your God—the Lord will send fearful plagues on you and your descendants, harsh and prolonged disasters, and severe and lingering illnesses. He will bring on

---

[lxxx] Sanctification, put simply, is to be made holy or set apart for God's use.

you all the <u>diseases</u> of Egypt that you dreaded, and <mark>they will cling to you</mark>. The Lord will also bring on you <u>every kind of sickness</u> and disaster not recorded in this Book of the Law, until you are destroyed.

There the Lord will give you an <u>anxious mind</u>, <u>eyes weary with longing</u>, and a <u>despairing heart</u>. You will live in constant suspense, <u>filled with dread</u> both night and day, never sure of your life. In the morning you will say, "If only it were evening!" and in the evening, "If only it were morning!"...This day I call the heavens and the earth as witnesses against you that I have set before you life and death, blessings and curses. Now choose life, so that you and your children may live and that you may love the Lord your God, listen to his voice, and hold fast to him. <u>For the Lord is your life</u>, and he will give you many years in the land he swore to give to your fathers, Abraham, Isaac, and Jacob.[lxxxi]

Wow! I am sure you agree; that seems harsh! After reading the many types of illnesses and areas of the body that God might afflict because of sin, we must call into question the idea that pain and disease largely arise from purely physical causes. That covenant describes everything from bacterial or viral diseases to cancer and psychological disorders. That is not to say that all of the illnesses listed are always the result of God's discipline for sin but only that they could have been under the covenant of the law.

Did you also notice the four highlighted references emphatically stating that the individuals stricken because of sin will not be cured? Why? It is not because those illnesses could not be cured, but that God would choose to block the way to healing when they persisted in sin. Such a possibility must resonate with all of those who endlessly pursue new and different doctors, treatments, pills, special diets and so on. Perhaps the reason none of those things have proven effective stems

---

[lxxxi] Deuteronomy 28:15, 21,22,27.28,35,59-61; 30:19-20.

from the fact that God Almighty has determined to stand in the way until repentance comes.

The question that arises, however, is whether or not the new covenant of grace, ushered in by Jesus,[lxxxii] eliminated the use of physical, mental and emotional illnesses as a curse for sin? Ahh, here semantics are crucial. For all of those under the blood of Christ, there is no condemnation because Jesus became the curse for us. Therefore, we do not fear the wrath or punishment of God.

However, I did discover and now share with you that the New Testament does carry over the teaching that God still uses illness as a tool for sanctifying His children. Therein lies our next biblical principle of health: **Illness is often a tool of discipline used by the loving Heavenly Father to sanctify His children**.

The Difference Between Discipline & Punishment

If you happened to grow up with a cruel or abusive parent, it might be difficult to differentiate between discipline and punishment. Understanding the difference is important when considering God's use of illness as a means of discipline. According to Merriam Webster's Dictionary, "punishment" is *suffering, pain, or loss that serves as retribution*.[48] Notice the striking difference between that and the definition of "discipline"--*training that corrects, molds, or perfects the mental faculties or moral character*.[49]

God, the Father, is not cruel but abounding in love. As evidence of this fact, Jesus, God's own perfect Son, suffered in our place the wrath or punishment of His Father for our sins. Jesus was the sinless, sacrificial lamb who shed His blood and died on the cross so that a holy God's requirement for justice could be met. *God made him who had no sin to be sin for us*[lxxxiii] and by doing so brought salvation from the

---

[lxxxii] Luke 4:19-21
[lxxxiii] 2 Corinthians 5:21

penalty of sin for all who would put their faith in Jesus as their Lord and Savior.

Many people hope being good, church attendance or membership, and other selfless acts might be enough to satisfy God and win them entrance into heaven. They are tragically mistaken. Isaiah 64:6 says, *All of us have become like one who is unclean, and all our righteous acts are like filthy rags.* Salvation is by grace alone, not by works.[lxxxiv] The Father loves everyone unfailingly, but only one thing satisfies Him--the blood payment of Jesus for sin. That and that alone satisfies completely.

If you have never trusted in Christ alone for salvation, then you do not fall under the blood of Christ and will one day face the eternal wrath of God for your sins. If you have yet to trust Christ, do not let another minute go by without doing so. You can stop right now and pray. Tell God that you are a sinner, and you believe that Jesus died in your place and rose from the dead three days later. Simple faith in Jesus saves you![lxxxv] Make sure to tell someone about your decision and begin reading the Bible. The book of Luke and Galatians are great New Testament books to start reading.

If you have trusted in Jesus Christ's work at the cross on your behalf, then you will never come under the wrath or punishment of God. However, just as good parents diligently discipline their children out of a loving desire to see them thriving in life, so also the heavenly Father disciplines His children. Unlike what some imagine, God does not expectantly wait with a stash of lightning bolts to strike us down when we make a mistake. Psalm 103:10 says that *He does not treat us as our sins deserve.* He will, however, carefully discipline His children when they persistently cling to sin. This discipline is not cruel, nor is it meant to punish but rather to restore a wayward child to the loving Father.

[lxxxiv] Ephesians 2:8-9
[lxxxv] "Believe in the Lord Jesus, and you will be saved." Acts 16:31

Sanctification

Let us consider two New Testament passages from 1 Thessalonians that speak of the sanctification from sin that God brings to pass in every one of His children.

- *For this is the will of God, your sanctification: that you abstain from sexual immorality; that each one of you know how to control his own body in holiness and honor, not in the passion of lust like the Gentiles who do not know God; that no one transgress and wrong his brother in this matter, because the Lord is an avenger in all these things, as we told you beforehand and solemnly warned you. For God has not called us for impurity, but in holiness.* (4:3-7 ESV)

- *May God himself, the God of peace, sanctify you through and through. May your whole spirit, soul and body be kept blameless at the coming of our Lord Jesus Christ. The one who calls you is faithful, and he will do it.* (5:23)

If you are astute, you may have noticed that, although these passages speak of sanctification from sin and a warning of discipline when necessary to bring that about, they do not specifically mention illness. However, a very stern warning to Christians by the Apostle Paul in 1 Corinthians 10:6-12 does and makes three direct connections between the discipline of the LORD at the time of the covenant of the law (blessings and curses) and the current time of grace.

> *Now these things occurred as examples to keep us from setting our hearts on evil things as they did. Do not be idolaters, as some of them were; as it is written: "The people sat down to eat and drink and got up to indulge in revelry." We should not commit sexual immorality, as some of them did—and in one day twenty-three thousand of them died. We should not test Christ, as some of them did—and were killed by snakes. And do not grumble, as some of them did—and were killed by the destroying angel. These things happened to them as examples and were*

written down as warnings for us, on whom the culmination of the ages has come. So, if you think you are standing firm, be careful that you don't fall!

We must not ignore such a strong warning. In the first of Paul's three examples, he quotes from Exodus 32:4, which tells of how the Israelites worshiped a golden calf and indulged in revelry.[lxxxvi] The verses in 1 Corinthians tell us the specific number killed by plague as a result of that sin--23,000. Paul's second reference mentions the time described in Numbers 21:4-9 when the Israelites complained against Moses and God for their hardships in the desert and were then poisoned by snakes. The third references Numbers 14 when the spies brought back a bad report of the Promised Land and caused the people to grumble once again against their Savior's provision. The spies who brought the bad report died of a plague, according to verse thirty-seven, which Paul refers to in 1 Corinthians as the destroying angel. As a result, all of those twenty years or older would die untimely deaths before God would finally lead His people into the Promised Land.[lxxxvii]

Now, I agree; Paul's words seem severe, but since he did give the warning so that God's people might live, what should be our response? I responded by seriously contemplating whether or not God was using my allergies to draw me to repentance. I will share the details of the healing that followed my repentance in the next chapter. My heart's desire is for others to know true and complete healing as well.

[lxxxvi] Exodus 32:4-6 &35 *He took what they handed him and made it into an idol cast in the shape of a calf, fashioning it with a tool. Then they said, "These are your gods, Israel, who brought you up out of Egypt." When Aaron saw this, he built an altar in front of the calf and announced, "Tomorrow there will be a festival to the Lord." So the next day the people rose early and sacrificed burnt offerings and presented fellowship offerings. Afterward they sat down to eat and drink and got up to indulge in revelry... And the Lord struck the people with **a plague** because of what they did with the calf Aaron had made.*

[lxxxvii] Numbers 14:26-30 & 37

Proper Fear

Most Christians know the story of Moses receiving the ten commandments on Mount Sinai and the Israelites disgraceful worship of the golden calf while their leader tarried on the mountain. Many times, I have read and even deeply studied this story from Exodus, but as I worked on this chapter, I noticed something that I had never reflected on previously.

God told Moses to have the people consecrate themselves and to be ready for the Lord's appearance on the mountain. The LORD established specific limits but instructed the people to come to the foot of the mountain so that they might personally witness God's power and hear for themselves the Almighty speaking the law to Moses.[lxxxviii] After a short time of this, the LORD told Moses to go back down to speak to the people who had chosen to move "a distance" from the mountain.[lxxxix] As it turns out, the terrified people forfeited their front-row seats and instead pleaded with Moses to speak to them for God but not to have Him speak directly to them.

Their wise leader responded with an incredibly profound statement: *Do not be afraid. God has come to test you, so that the fear of God will be with you to keep you from sinning.*[xc]

At first reading, it seems odd for Moses to tell them that they should not be afraid but then tell them to fear God. So, what was he saying? God desired for His people to be in His presence and wanted to reveal Himself directly to them; therefore, they had no reason to fear that God might harm them. God's character is not capricious. He does not say one thing and do another. However, God did intend for the dramatic display of His power on the mountain to be a strong reminder that fear of such a powerful God should keep them from sin.

So many people today fear the wrong things. We fear our circumstances (like the Israelites when Mt. Sinai quaked), as though

---

[lxxxviii] Exodus 19:10-19
[lxxxix] Exodus 20:18
[xc] Exodus 20:20

God lacks control or is not good and loving. Unfortunately, few today fear God for the reason they should--that a holy, omnipotent God who loves His children still disciplines for sin, and often does so specifically through physical suffering. Proverbs 14:27 says, *The fear of the Lord is a fountain of life, turning a person from the snares of death.* His desire is not to curse or harm His children but to save them from death. Therefore, illness should be like a warning light, meant to alert us to unrepented patterns of sin that must be addressed so that life can abound.

Practical Application

Do you have ongoing physical, mental, or emotional symptoms, whether diagnosed or undiagnosed, managed or unmanaged, treated or untreated? Have you sought various means to get better, all to no avail? Have you prayed for healing and remained the same or even worsened over time? I do not presume to know the reason for any individual's lingering health problems. I only know that Scripture clearly indicates that God does often use illness as a means of discipline. Therefore, with great love in my heart for those who suffer, I urge anyone who answers "yes" to one of the questions above to honestly consider the possibility that those symptoms stem from the Lord's discipline.

Why should God allow healing if His people refuse to repent? Do not forget, the blood of forgiveness must precede the oil of healing. Is the pleasure of any sin, including your pride, worth the constant struggle, turmoil, expense, and suffering that poor health inflicts? Is holding on to any sin worth dying for? Your heavenly Father loves you too much to let you remain separated from His fellowship indefinitely. If the root of your illness is sin and the Father intends to use illness to restore you, then you will not get better until repentance or heaven comes.

Has the Lord already prompted your heart about a pattern of sin in your life in which you continue to indulge? Comparing ourselves to others is not helpful. We stand before God, not an unrighteous world. Ask the Lord to break your heart over your sin so that you might truly repent and turn from it.

Often, though, people have chronic symptoms and illness but are unaware of any pattern of sin. *The heart is deceitful above all things, and desperately wicked: who can know it?* says Jeremiah 17:9 (KJV). That is why I encourage you to simply begin asking the Lord daily to search your heart and reveal to you if there is a sin issue that has brought about the Father's discipline through illness. Fasting might also be advisable.[xci] God will faithfully show you, just as He did me if your symptoms exist because of a pattern of sinful behavior or thought. The prompting of the Holy Spirit, especially while you spend time in God's Word, will bring revelation.

Something I found helpful when I began asking the Lord to search my heart was to write 1 Timothy 2:25-26 as a personalized prayer on a notecard. Here it is with the pronouns personalized:

God, grant me repentance leading me to a knowledge of the truth that I may come to my senses and escape from the trap of the devil, who has taken me captive to do his will.

If God does reveal a pattern of sin to you, confess it (own up to it) and turn away from it. Often our sin damages others, and therefore the need may exist to ask others for forgiveness as well. If the sin lies solely in wrong thinking or attitudes, then confess it and begin taking *captive every thought to make it obedient to Christ.*[xcii] You may also need to ask someone to hold you accountable and to pray for you to withstand the temptations of the evil one. Finally, Paul's advice will serve you well--*But put on the Lord Jesus Christ, and make no provision for the flesh, to gratify its desires* (ESV).[xciii] Burn whatever

---

[xci] For more information on fasting, see Appendix H.
[xcii] 2 Corinthians 10:5
[xciii] Romans 13:14 Ephesians 4:27

bridges need burning to rid yourself of the pattern of sin that ensnares and take whatever action, no matter how humbling it might be, to repent. Be ruthless with your sin. Your heart and your health are at stake!

However, if your illness does not come from the Father's discipline, He will give you peace in that regard. Until then, it is wise to continue to pray and seek God on the matter. In the next chapter, I will focus on God's promise for healing when one truly repents. God's desire is not to leave us in sin and discipline but to restore us fully. Read on!

Biblical Principle: *Illness is often a tool of discipline used by a loving Heavenly Father to sanctify His children.*

Call to Action: *If you are ill, ask the Lord to search your heart and reveal to you any unrepented sin or patterns of sin in your life so that you might repent.*

CHAPTER 11

Repentance Brings Healing

Repent, then, and turn to God, so that your sins may be wiped out, that times of refreshing may come from the Lord. Acts 3:19

After I came to understand the biblical connection between sin and illness, I felt overwhelmed and yet determined to discover if those teachings applied to my abundance of allergies. Suddenly, the offense to my pride at such a possibility mattered very little. I just wanted to be well and not propped up by frequent "treatments." As a result, I desperately wanted God to reveal any areas of sin in my life that might have made necessary God's discipline. One problem existed. I was blind to the deception of my heart, and no sin came readily to mind. I recalled that the Bible speaks of praying for God to search our hearts,[xciv] so I began to do just that. I encourage you to do the same. I simply began praying daily that God would search my heart and reveal to me any sin that He found therein.

For two weeks I prayed along those lines. Faithfully, God answered and moved in my heart so that I might confess my sins to the great High Priest, Jesus, as well as to whomever I might have wronged. Each day brought new things to light. Although this proved humbling

---

[xciv] Romans 8:27, 1 Chronicles 28:9, Psalm 139:23, & Jeremiah 17:10

to me, it became almost comical to my son. After some days of seeking his forgiveness for various things from the past, he would hear me launch into yet another tearful apology and start to laugh. "Mom, it's ok," he would say. "Yes, I forgive you." Regardless of how uncomfortable the process made me or others, I continued to repent humbly of anything the Lord brought to my attention.

I could not believe all the sins that I had allowed to go unnoticed through the years or even managed to justify in my self-righteousness. Like a long shower after a weekend of primitive camping, my weeks of repentance left me feeling clean and refreshed. Although my initial motivation came from my new understanding of the biblical principle that **true repentance leads to healing from illness due to sin**, in the process, God transformed my heart.

When God did not call to my mind any further areas in need of repentance, I got down on my knees and prayed according to my understanding that repentance leads to healing. "Lord, I have repented of all that you have revealed to me. Now, if I understand your Word correctly, you have promised to heal me. Please heal me of all my allergies."

God responded to my heart's desire for holiness, even though I was still far from attaining the goal and mercifully began the process of healing. The immediate and definitive change occurred following my prayer for healing; I no longer tested "allergic" to anything whatsoever. The constant reactions to everything subsided, and I was never again treated through Applied Kinesiology for anything.

I will mention, though, that I had developed quite a fear of food because of the pain the previous reactions had created. My negative physical responses to that fear diminished as I used God's Word to transform my mind and make eating pleasurable once again. (I will address this more in chapter 18 on nutrition.)

Still not recognizing AK as a sin though, I continued using those practices in an attempt to help others. Little did I know, but my long-suffering Savior had just begun to peel back the veil and reveal to me strong evidence of the demonic forces at work in Applied Kinesiology (more on that in chapter 17).

Repentance Leads to Healing

My story of complete healing, no matter how unusual each episode was, highlights the power of God's Word. First, His Word bound up my broken heart by transforming my understanding of the limitless love of God, and as a result, all my hormone issues were healed. Then, the Bible spoke to me of my self-righteousness and critical spirit and brought repentance that allowed God to heal me of my "allergies." Finally, God's Word transformed my thought patterns of despair and healed me of chronic depression.

Psalm 107:20 says it well: *He sent out his Word and healed them. He rescued them from the grave.* Wow! Because Christians often minimize their exposure to the Bible, they forfeit the healing power of the Word. Let me put it in a different way. Jesus, the Logos or Word as John calls Him, often simply spoke whenever He healed people. His Word, God's Word, is power! According to Scripture, a significant means of healing comes from the Word of God, and therefore, not knowing and following it results in people who perish. If only the sick would seek after God through His Word with the same fervency that they seek for answers from the medical establishment, traditional or otherwise. That is why this book is chock-full of Scripture. My words and thoughts have no power, but God's Word does!

In the last chapter, I shared with you the biblical principle that illness is often a tool of discipline by a loving Heavenly Father to sanctify His children. In this chapter, I wish to take that principle a step further and establish that when God uses illness as a means of discipline, the purpose is to bring His children to a place of repentance so that He might then heal them completely. In our sinfulness, we might not notice that we have drifted from God or even care enough to turn from our sin. However, the unpleasantness of illness effectively grabs our attention.

The reason for discipline, after all, is NOT to punish but to bring about change. Unfortunately, the modern Christian often fails to connect illness with God's discipline. As a result, people pray for healing without considering the possible need for repentance that must precede God's work of healing from illness due to sin. Do you recall the ceremony of cleansing from Leviticus 14 that was discussed in chapter 8 of this book? If you remember, the placement of the blood of sanctification on the right earlobe, right thumb, and right big toe preceded the placing of the oil of healing/blessing. Healing follows cleansing from sin, not the other way around.

God Responds to a Repentant Heart

Among the biblical kings, the good king Asa stands out against a backdrop of great wickedness by his many predecessors. As we discussed in chapter two, King Asa did all he could to rid the land of pagan worship, including going against his own grandmother. The Bible speaks highly of how he diligently sought the Lord. However, despite his faithful service to God, Asa made one mistake. He chose to figure out a solution to a problem by man's wisdom rather than seeking God for direction. Rather than repenting when confronted with God's displeasure, King Asa became angry and stubborn. Yes, even godly individuals fall prey to their sin nature.

As we consider the biblical teaching that repentance leads to healing, I feel we must also address a reasonable sounding argument that arises when considering the many people who are sick, who truly love the Lord and live godly lives. Surely the fact that godly people are sick and not healed indicates their illness must not be the result of God's discipline. The story of King Asa shows that such an assumption might prove false. Instead, God severely disciplined the godly king with an illness for what seems to us a minor sin. Perhaps the king's greater knowledge of God and responsibility as His representative before others led to a higher standard. *From everyone who has been given much, much will be demanded; and from the one who has been entrusted with much, much more will be asked.*[xcv]

Unlike King Asa who rebelled against God's discipline rather than repenting and eventually died of his illness, Hezekiah did turn to the Lord when he was deathly ill. The Bible does not tell us why the godly king became sick, but in his own prayer following that illness, he speaks of his sin. When Isaiah told him of his impending death, the king with a tender heart immediately repented and tearfully pleaded with the Lord for healing. God, always faithful and merciful, immediately sent Isaiah back into Hezekiah's chambers with medicinal instructions and promises of complete healing. Upon recovering his health, the good king prayed the following words out of a thankful heart.

> *You restored me to health and let me live. Surely it was for my benefit that I suffered such anguish. In your love you kept me from the pit of destruction; you have put all my sins behind your back. For the grave cannot praise you, death cannot sing your praise.* (Isaiah 38:16b-18)

A Biblical Duo--Forgiveness & Healing

Consider a story found in Acts chapter three that describes Peter's healing of a lame man. Just imagine the shocked reaction of the people present! This man, crippled from birth, had for many years been carried daily to the entrance of the temple courts to beg for a living. When Peter healed him, the people witnessed this familiar lame man suddenly jumping around and praising God. The healing, of course, gave Peter a fantastic opportunity for a sermon to the ever-growing and inquisitive crowd that gathered around the apostle and his new convert. Peter explained the healing to them by declaring, ***Repent, then, and***

[xcv] Luke 12:48

turn to God, so that your sins may be wiped out, that times of refreshing may come from the Lord.[xcvi]

What does repentance have to do with healing? According to Peter's message, repentance brings two benefits--the forgiveness of sins AND *times of refreshing*. Understanding this duo is key. In the Greek, "refreshed" means "recovery of breath."[50] This picturesque word only shows up one other time in the Bible. In 2 Timothy 1:16, Paul speaks of how Onesiphorus "refreshed" the weary missionary many times. Consider how the beaten and battered apostle, who frequently went without proper care and who suffered reproach and stress at every turn, might need refreshment. Surely, Paul's need encompassed spirit, soul, and body.

Consider also that without breath life ceases. Genesis 2:7, *And the Lord God formed man of the dust of the ground, and breathed into his nostrils the breath of life; and man became a living soul* (KJV). The agent of life throughout the Bible is the Spirit, which literally means *breath* (Hebrew--*ruach*). The Breath breathes life into lifeless things.[xcvii] So, Peter ties repentance to healing (the recovery of breath) by using the word refreshing.

The context of "refreshed" in the New Testament indicates a refreshing of the whole person--spirit, soul, and body. Furthermore, based on the specific context of the lame man's healing and the Gospel message found in Peter's sermon, his intended meaning of "times of refreshing" must be the healing of the whole man. God first deals with the heart of sin (*that your sins may be wiped out*) and then follows with a time of recovering your breath—healing spirit, soul, and body.

When we get sick, our thoughts understandably center on the need for physical wellness, but God, on our behalf, considers our situation comprehensively. Although He cares much about the physical body, He desires to restore the whole person--spirit, soul, and body. Remember--out of the heart (soul and spirit) flows life. Abundant life

---

[xcvi] Acts 3:19
[xcvii] i.e., Genesis 2:7, 6:17, 7:15 & 22, Ezekiel 37:5-10, Romans 8:11

does not come with mere physical wellness, but instead when the heart finds peace. Do you need to recover your breath, to be refreshed in spirit, soul, and body? According to Acts 3:19, repentance leads to the forgiveness of sins AND a refreshing of your whole person. What a beautiful promise!

The psalmist, King David, also portrays the biblical duo of forgiveness and healing in Psalm 103:3. *Praise the LORD, O my soul, and forget not all his benefits. He forgives all my sins and heals all my diseases.* This remarkably promises both forgiveness and healing in the same breath! As we continue reading in the same passage, verse twelve powerfully shows the completeness of this forgiveness—*As far as the east is from the west, so far has he removed our transgressions from us.*

If you question the literal truth of the first benefit--that God forgives ALL your sins--verse twelve of the chapter leaves no room for doubt. However, is this complete forgiveness of sins automatic for all people? No. Although God, on the basis of Christ's shed blood, freely gives the benefit of complete forgiveness to all people for all sin, not all recognize their need and turn to God in faith. Therefore, availability may not equal reality.

Now consider the second benefit of Psalm 103:3: *heals all my diseases.* It is noteworthy that the wording of that phrase mirrors *forgives all my sins.* Just as the benefit of the forgiveness for all sins exists for all but only become a reality for those who receive it according to God's terms, so too is the case with healing.

I have wrestled much with this verse. Does it indeed promise the healing of all diseases in this life? Many would understandably say *no*, that it refers to eternal healing. Such an interpretation certainly aligns well with the reality that many people go to their graves with some conditions, such as serious injuries or serious disabilities with which people are born. After much study, I have come to believe another interpretation.

As I have already shown from Scripture, we know biblically that not all illnesses, disabilities, or injuries are due to sin. The dual nature of these two promises—for forgiveness and healing indicates that IF a disease is due to sin, God promises BOTH forgiveness AND healing following repentance from the pattern of sin that brought the Father's discipline through illness. Therefore, healing from ALL diseases is to be understood in the context of all diseases brought about by sin.

Think of it this way. Could the man born blind be healed sooner had he or his parents repented of sin? No. Because Jesus made it clear the cause of illness and the reason for it when he said in John 9:3: *"Neither this man nor his parents sinned," said Jesus, "but this happened so that the works of God might be displayed in him.* His healing had nothing to do with repentance.

Additionally, consider Job. We also know that his skin disease and tremendous physical suffering was a spiritual attack that God allowed that was in no way due to sin. So, again I ask: Could Job have been healed sooner if he had repented or if he just had enough faith. Certainly not!

If we put all of this together, we can draw several conclusions. In the two instances of the man born blind and Job, we see that not all disease is due to God's discipline, nor is all healing due to repentance. But, if we return to our consideration of the meaning of the promises in Psalm 103:3 to forgive all our sins and heal all our diseases, as well as the clear statement from Isaiah and Peter that we are healed by His wounds, then we realize the pairing of sin and illness is critical to rightly dividing the true meaning. When sin is the cause of disease, then, provision by Jesus' blood brings the forgiveness of that sin and His stripes bring healing.

We do not question the forgiveness of *all* of our sins; neither should we doubt the promise of healing David speaks of under the inspiration of the Holy Spirit. However, one further point is needed. We must not overlook the order of the forgiveness/healing duo in both Acts 3:19 and Psalm 103:3--first comes repentance from sin and then comes complete refreshment/healing.

The Promise of Hebrews 12:11-13

Let us also consider Hebrews twelve, which is entirely devoted to explaining how our loving, heavenly Father disciplines His children for their good, and why we should not despise that discipline. To grasp fully this chapter's culminating promise that healing follows repentance, one must notice that the author of Hebrews specifically quotes Proverbs 3:11-12 and 4:26. In fact, upon studying Hebrews twelve, it becomes abundantly clear that this chapter intends to not merely quote snippets from Proverbs three and four but to mirror it entirely.

Therefore, by looking back to the Old Testament text, we gain further insight into chapter twelve. In Proverbs three and four, Solomon speaks specifically of health and life twelve times! The metaphor of the path of life permeates both chapters. Interwoven with God's promises for health while walking the path of life are warnings against disobedience and instruction not to despise God's discipline should it prove necessary.

With that context in mind, let us now consider Hebrews 12:9-13, taking note of the references to life, peace, and healing.

> *Moreover, we have all had human fathers who disciplined us, and we respected them for it. How much more should we <u>submit to the Father of spirits and live</u>! They disciplined us for a little while as they thought best; but God disciplines us for our good, in order that we may share in his holiness. No discipline seems pleasant at the time, <u>but painful. Later on,</u> however, it produces a harvest of <u>righteousness and peace</u> for those who have been trained by it. Therefore, strengthen your feeble arms and weak knees. "Make level paths for your feet," so that the lame may not be disabled, <u>but rather healed.</u>*

God's heart is for His children to walk in the tremendous blessing of fellowship with the Father, but sin alters that sweet communion. Just as Acts 3:19 speaks of repentance leading to forgiveness of sins and then refreshing, so the verses in Hebrews refer first to a *harvest of righteousness and peace* that then culminates in healing. Discipline is not an end in itself, but a means to bring about the restoration of the whole man--complete healing.

A Painful Personal Reminder

As I prepared to write these chapters, God gave me an excruciating reminder that the Father disciplines for sin, and repentance leads to healing. Because I live for close fellowship with my Savior but also fear His power to lovingly but painfully discipline for sin, I attempt to keep short accounts with Him. However, like everyone, I am susceptible to the temptations of the flesh and the heart's willingness to be deceived. For quite some time, I knew that I frequently walked too close to a particular God-established boundary. My attempt at walking the line meant that I often could not distinguish between when I managed to remain on the right side, and when I had crossed over it. I justified the pattern of behavior by convincing myself that I never truly crossed the line. Despite my internal justifications, I had no peace.

I am ashamed to say that on one particular occasion I strongly felt the Lord's caution in this area but blatantly chose to ignore it. Two or three days later I began having pain in my low back. The pain then escalated to unbearable proportions over the next several days. After several days of attempting to manage the pain with narcotic pain relievers left-over from a previous injury, I finally went to the emergency room with my back muscles in torturous spasms. It took Morphine and two other powerful drugs to quiet my cries. The following day I broke out in the characteristic rash of Shingles and spent the next two weeks with an excruciating reminder that my Heavenly Father loves me too much to allow me to continue walking in sin.

I felt the powerful truth of Hebrews 12:11 when it says, *No discipline seems pleasant at the time, but painful. Later on, however, it produces a harvest of righteousness and peace for those who have been trained by it.* I knew without a doubt that my case of Shingles was brought on as a much-deserved act of discipline. Would I allow myself to be "trained by it" or would I respond with anger? Like Hezekiah, my heart broke over my pattern of sin. I was finally ready to repent, not only for crossing the line but for walking that line for so long. Through my pain and sickness, God restored my heart to righteousness and therefore, peace in an area that had been in turmoil for far too long.

Although relieved to once again be truly at peace with my Savior, I cannot adequately describe the fear I felt that God might leave me in that physical state of pain. Many people with Shingles develop lingering nerve pain that lasts for years or never goes away. I knew I deserved no less. However, I also knew that Scripture teaches that God did not discipline me to be cruel, but to bring me to repentance so that I might be healed--spirit, soul, and body.

The verses in Ezekiel 18:30-32 came to mind and brought reassurance to my terrified heart.

> *Repent! Turn away from all your offenses; then sin will not be your downfall. Rid yourselves of all the offenses you have committed, and get a new heart and a new spirit. Why will you die, people of Israel? For I take no pleasure in the death of anyone, declares the Sovereign Lord. Repent and live!*

With those promises in mind, I pleaded for God's mercy and complete healing. The illness, however, continued unabated. I began to waver in my faith as fear attempted to take hold. "Perhaps I have misunderstood God's promise that with repentance comes healing," I thought. Anxiousness mounted as memories of twenty years of living with daily pain resurfaced and tormented my mind.

On such a morning, I again fretfully pleaded for mercy and healing. The phrase from Hebrews 12:11, *later on, however, it produces*... came to mind, indicating that the benefit of healing might not come right away. I sensed the Lord impressing on me to wait and trust. I did not need to keep pleading for healing; I simply needed to wait and trust for the "later on."

With that assurance in mind, a measure of peace returned despite the pain's continuance. Thankfully, in two days' time, I improved significantly and within another week considered myself 90% better. The remaining twinges of pain continued to improve over the next two weeks and served as a gentle reminder, a tool for training, if you will, to continue walking in righteousness. Within another week or two, even the lingering nerve sensitivity disappeared. The "later on" had come, and God once again showed Himself to be faithful to His promises. Praise be to God!

A Door of Hope

To our human and modern way of thinking, causing someone to suffer pain is cruel. Many parents will not even spank their children appropriately because they view it as a cruel form of discipline. My husband and I were not of that mindset. Do not get me wrong. I hated to spank our son, but I loved seeing the change in heart it brought about and the fruit of happiness it produced in the end. It is usually quite easy to tell a child who gets appropriately spanked from one who does not, not only by the vast difference in overall behavior but in their apparent enjoyment of life. As odd as it might seem, the carefully disciplined child seems to be more able to enjoy his parents and vice versa. That certainly proved true of our son.

Similarly, God knows that left to our own devices, we make a wreck of things, which takes us out of sweet fellowship with Him and makes life less enjoyable. Because God is a loving Father, He desires that His children have an abundant life. If temporary pain will bring that to pass, it is well worth it.

Hosea prophesied how God intended to discipline the rebellious nation of Israel. In chapter two of Hosea, God speaks of repeatedly blocking the way and bringing hardship to His children for one purpose--that in their time of trouble they would hear His voice and turn back to Him. *Therefore, I am now going to allure her; I will lead her into the <u>wilderness</u> and speak tenderly to her. There <u>I will</u> give her back her vineyards and will make the Valley of <u>Achor</u> a door of hope.*[xcviii]

The Hebrew meaning of the keywords in this passage serves to emphasize the history of the Valley of Achor and provides a powerful metaphor. "Achor" means "trouble." The word "wilderness" is used synonymously in Scripture with the desert, which evokes endless pictures of harsh barrenness. The Valley of Achor received the name "trouble" because it was the location where God dealt severely with the sin of an Israelite man named Achan.

Joshua 6:18-19 tells how God instructed the Israelites that, upon defeating Jericho, everything in the city should remain as the Lord's and not be taken for personal plunder. Any disobedience in the matter would result in disaster for all of Israel. Achan, however, failed to resist the lure of treasure and took some for himself, thinking no one would find out about the carefully hidden items in his tent. God knew, though, and true to His promise, Israel suffered defeat in their next battle at Ai with the loss of many lives. Through this unexpected loss, God brought to Joshua's attention the sin of Achan. Once made known, the Judge of all the earth dealt with Achan's sin abruptly and completely so as to restore Israel once again to a right walk with Himself.

With the context of that story in mind, we can more rightly understand what God desires to communicate through the prophet Hosea. Sometimes God lovingly leads His children into a valley of suffering (*the wilderness*) so that repentance might come. Then, what was lost (*her vineyards*-- representative of blessing) can once again be restored. In that way, God transforms the valley of trouble into *a door of hope.*

[xcviii] Hosea 2:14-15

Has God lured you into the wilderness of suffering so that you might more readily listen to the tender voice of His Word? It is a question worth considering because therein just might be your door of hope.

Cry out to God as the psalmist does. Have mercy *on me, LORD; heal me, for I have sinned against you* (Psalm 41:4). Then, the Lord, who does not lie, will act.

Biblical Principle: *True repentance leads to healing from illness due to sin.*

Call to Action: *If God has called to mind any areas needing repentance, confess that sin. When you no longer sense the Spirit's conviction, ask God to heal you in light of the promises stated in His Word. Then, patiently wait in trust for the "later on" when the healing will come (Hebrews 12:11).*

CHAPTER 12

His Wounds--Our Healing

"He himself bore our sins" in his body on the cross, so that we might die to sins and live for righteousness; "by his wounds you have been healed." 1 Peter 2:24

During a discussion time in a Bible study, a man described how he felt like a hypocrite when asked to pray for healing while visiting someone in the hospital. Having years earlier lost his wife to cancer, he went on to insist that Christians do not actually believe God is going to heal because no one truly gets healed. Sensing that God would call me to account if I failed to share the healing work He had done in me, I humbly shared my story. However, this incident illustrates the thinking of many in Christendom and, if we are honest, for good reason.

I am fully aware of the many Christians who deal with plaguing symptoms, chronic illnesses, and significant pain and the rarity of notable healings. As I have wrestled with aligning what appears to be the reality of poor health in a fallen world with the teachings in Scripture on healing, I am aware of three options to explain the dichotomy. The first option is the interpretation many in Christianity have come to, which is that the Bible never promises physical healing in this life but only in the next. The second option is the interpretation of the more charismatic branch of Christianity, which is that when healing has not come, the reason rests solely in the individual's lack of faith. A third option is that the Word of God does promise physical healing from disease in this life but that numerous factors impact the fulfillment of that promise. I find that people tend to want a black and white answer—either that God will heal, or we cannot expect healing until the next life; when, instead, I have come to understand through much study that the biblical answer is far more complex and beautiful.

As previously discussed, the heart as the wellspring of life is one of those beautiful complexities that greatly influences the development of and recovery from illness. Ignore this God-created aspect of humanity and healing will likely remain elusive. Additionally, I have written of the biblical teaching that the loving Father often disciplines His children through illness. When such is the case, our next biblical principle of health and healing comes into play: **Jesus' suffering at the cross conquered the curse of the flesh (death), making provision through sanctification so that we can be healed**. Jesus did it all, and the gracious, heavenly Father has revealed His magnificent plan from Genesis to Revelation for all who will listen.

Why a Death of Great Suffering?

The dual nature of sin and illness, as well as repentance and healing are profound themes seen throughout the Bible. The direct connection between sin and death began in the Garden, and so it should come as no surprise that God, as our healer, made provision for both physical and spiritual healing through the cross. *By his wounds we are healed.*[xcix]

Some time ago, a thought occurred to me while studying Christ's work at the cross: *I knew why Jesus had to die, but why was it necessary for him to die in such a tortuous manner?* Shortly before

---

[xcix] Isaiah 53:5

Judas' betrayal, Jesus told His disciples quite specifically in Matthew 16:21 that three things must happen to Him: He must suffer, be killed, and be raised from the dead. We recognize that death and resurrection were necessary, but why must He also have suffered?[c]

I recall seeing Mel Gibson's movie, "The Passion of the Christ," in a theater some years ago. Watching that portrayal of Jesus' suffering made me physically ill. Even now, as I write this, tears flow at the thought of the incredible suffering my precious Savior endured on my account. Following the movie, I went home and reread, quite carefully, the biblical accounts to determine if the movie had in any way exaggerated the length and extent of Jesus' suffering. Sadly, it did not.

A permanent, sinless, blood sacrifice had to be made to satisfy God's justice on account of man's sin. However, if that was all that was needed, surely the method of death could have been an abrupt slaying that included the shedding of Jesus' blood. Why did the loving Father allow the beatings and a torturous, prolonged method of execution for His Son? If all that was necessary was death and resurrection, allowing such a horrific death would have been terribly cruel of the Father. Indeed, I will show from an abundance of Scripture that one purpose for this grievous torment was so that Christ might suffer the curse of the flesh in our place, thereby making provision, not only for our atonement but also for our healing.

The LORD Made Jesus *Sick*

1 Peter 2:24 most succinctly states the accomplishment of Christ's suffering—*by his wounds you have been healed*. Peter quotes that phrase from the prophecy found in Isaiah 53, which vividly portrays the suffering of the Messiah. However, in our modern translations, we forfeit an incredible depth of meaning that Isaiah intended to be understood, tying illness and healing with the suffering of Christ. To

---

[c] Romans 4:24-25 *It will be counted to us who believe in him who raised from the dead Jesus our Lord, who was delivered up for our trespasses and raised for our justification.* (ESV)

regain this understanding, we need to do a bit of word study for two words. I will insert the Hebrew meaning in parenthesis.

> *Surely, he has borne our griefs and carried our sorrows; yet we esteemed him stricken, smitten by God, and afflicted. But he was pierced for our transgressions; he was crushed for our iniquities; upon him was the chastisement that brought us peace, and with his __wounds__* (stripes; a black and blue mark[51]) *we are healed.* (vs.4-5)

> *And they made his grave with the wicked and with a rich man in his death, although he had done no violence, and there was no deceit in his mouth. Yet it was the will of the Lord to crush him; he has __put him to grief__* (to make weak, sick, or diseased[52] vs. 9-10 ESV)

A few verses later, Isaiah makes a striking and very intentional choice of words when he describes the will of Yahweh. In the Hebrew language, there are ten different words for "grief," yet God chose the only one that specifically means sickness. That detail helps us see the deeper meaning behind Jesus' horrific death: He was *made sick* in our place so that we might be made whole—just as He carried our sins so that we might be forgiven.

Mark continues this same powerful imagery in the New Testament by using an unusual Greek word when he talks about disease. Instead of choosing from the many common words for illness or affliction, he uses the word *mastix*, which literally means "whip" or "scourge." He does this three times.

In one passage, Mark writes, *For he had healed many, so that those with __diseases__* (a whip, scourge) *were pushing forward to touch him.*[ci] The other two times Mark uses *mastix*, he is describing the woman who suffered from an issue of blood for eighteen years before

---

[ci] Mark 3:10

she touched Jesus and was healed. It raises a thoughtful question: Did Mark choose this word on purpose, following Isaiah's imagery, to connect the scourging Jesus would endure at the cross with the sickness He came to heal?

We Can Be Healed

To really understand what Peter is pointing to when he quotes Isaiah 53:5, we need to pay attention to something simple but powerful: the tense of the verbs. I know—grammar doesn't usually sound exciting. But stay with me, because this is actually one of those moments where the meaning comes alive.

Listen closely to the way the verse reads: ***But he WAS pierced for our transgressions, he WAS crushed for our iniquities; the punishment that brought us peace WAS upon him, and by his wounds we ARE healed.***[cii]

Notice what is happening there. The prophecy uses three verbs in the past tense. The first two—was pierced and was crushed—describe the once-and-for-all physical suffering and death of the Messiah. The third, also in the past tense, tells us that His punishment brought us peace. Those verbs send a clear message: the work of ending the separation between God and humanity is complete. Finished. It isn't ongoing. Jesus' death fully met God's requirement—period.

But then something changes. One part of the work of the cross continues, and you can see it in the sudden shift in tense: ***by his wounds we are healed.*** That phrase is not in the past or the future. It describes an ongoing state—something that is happening now. If it were meant only as a future promise, it would say "we will be healed." Instead, it speaks of a present, continuing reality.

That shift suggests healing isn't just a finished event in the past or a blessing reserved only for heaven someday. It's an ongoing benefit for the believer here and now.

[cii] Isaiah 53:5

Other passages seem to echo this same idea. Take Romans 8:11, for example: *And if the Spirit of him who raised Jesus from the dead is living in you, he who raised Christ from the dead will also give life to your <u>mortal</u> bodies because of his Spirit who lives in you.*

This verse sits in the middle of a longer section about how living according to the Spirit brings life and peace, while living according to the flesh leads to death. Even a quick reading makes it clear that Paul is talking about how we live in this present life, not only about something waiting for us in heaven.

The Two Elements of Communion

Another strong sign that the healing made available through Jesus' stripes, as described by both Peter and Isaiah, is meant for the here and now can be found in the sacrament of communion. The bread and the wine draw our attention to a two-part work that Jesus accomplished at the cross, yet this distinction is often overlooked.

Have you ever paused to ask why God established communion with two separate elements, the body and the blood? Is one simply repeating the meaning of the other? The answer is no. Each one points to a distinct aspect of the work of the cross: the forgiveness of sins through the blood, and the breaking of the curse of the flesh, which is death, making possible life for the body, which is healing.

The key passage that explains the practice of communion, 1 Corinthians 11:23–32, begins by carefully describing these two elements on their own. First comes the bread, which represents the body of Christ. Second comes the cup, which represents His blood.

1. *For I received from the Lord what I also delivered to you, that the Lord Jesus on the night when he was betrayed took <u>bread</u>, and when he had given thanks, he broke it, and said, "This is my <u>body</u>, which is for you. Do this in remembrance of me."* (ESV vs 23-24)

2. *In the same way also he took the <u>cup</u>, after supper, saying, "This cup is the new covenant in my <u>blood</u>. Do this, as often as you drink it, in remembrance of me."* (ESV v 25)

At this point, the apostle Paul begins to link the two elements together. In fact, he does this six times. Every time he refers to the bread or the body, he also includes the cup or the blood. At first, the repetition can seem unnecessary or even awkward, unless it is meant to highlight how distinct and yet inseparable these two components truly are. Notice how intentional Paul is in the way he writes.

For as often as you <u>eat this bread and drink the cup</u>, you proclaim the Lord's death until he comes. Whoever, therefore, <u>eats the bread or drinks the cup</u> of the Lord in an unworthy manner will be guilty concerning <u>the body and blood of the Lord</u>. Let a person examine himself, then, and so <u>eat of the bread and drink of the cup</u>. For anyone who <u>eats and drinks</u> without discerning the <u>body eats and drinks</u> judgment on himself. That is why many of you are weak and ill, and some have died. But if we judged ourselves truly, we would not be judged. But when we are judged by the Lord, we are disciplined so that we may not be condemned along with the world.
(ESV vs. 26-32)

Since this book is focused on a biblical understanding of health and healing, I need to draw special attention to the strong warning at the end of this passage. Paul makes it clear that believers are to deal with their sin before taking communion. He even specifies that the discipline that can follow a failure to examine oneself may take the form of weakness, illness, and in some cases, death.

To understand why such serious consequences are connected specifically to wrongly partaking of the body and blood of Christ, we need to look even deeper.

Understanding Flesh and Blood

Since Paul repeatedly distinguishes between the body and the blood of Christ, each part of communion must point to something unique. But what does each one represent? To answer that, we need to follow the thread of "flesh and blood" as it runs through Scripture.

Today, most people use the phrase "flesh and blood" simply to mean the physical parts that make up a living being. In that sense, the phrase means the same thing in God's Word. But in the Bible, flesh and blood also carry a spiritual meaning, which adds an important layer of depth.

There is no denying that the Bible places great emphasis on blood. Because of the vivid and sometimes gruesome way blood appears throughout Leviticus, and really throughout all of Scripture, its importance is hard to miss. The Levitical law repeatedly highlights the role of blood in the sacrifices made for sin. *For the life of a creature is in the blood, and I have given it to you to make atonement for yourselves on the altar; it is the blood that makes atonement for one's life.*[ciii]

The writer of Hebrews echoes this same theme when speaking about the blood of Jesus. *In fact, the law requires that nearly everything be cleansed with blood, and without the shedding of blood there is no forgiveness.*[civ]   From these passages, it becomes clear that while blood is physical, it also carries deep spiritual significance.

The meaning of "flesh," however, can be even more challenging. In both Hebrew and Greek, there is primarily one main word for flesh, and that single word carries both physical and spiritual meanings. [53] It refers to the physical body, including things like muscle, fat, and the body as a whole, but it also refers to the carnal or sin nature. In a way, using one word for both draws attention to how closely the Bible ties together the physical and spiritual meanings of the flesh.

To understand this connection, we need to go back to the Garden and the curse. When Adam and Eve sinned, death entered human flesh for the first time, just as God had warned. [cv] At that moment, two

---

[ciii] Leviticus 17:11
[civ] Hebrews 9:22
[cv] Genesis 2:17 & 3:19

problems came into existence, not just one. There was sin, which brought separation from God, and there was the curse, which brought death to all flesh. Justice needed to be satisfied, but death also needed to be overcome.

Moving forward to the time of Abraham, we encounter the covenant of circumcision, which may seem strange at first. God said, *You are to undergo circumcision, and it will be the sign of the covenant between me and you...My covenant in your flesh is to be an everlasting covenant.*[cvi]

Through this covenant, God promised that Abraham would become the father of many nations and that God Himself would be their God. This agreement was both literally and symbolically tied to the flesh, and it pointed ahead to the day when it would be fulfilled in Christ, in His flesh. Through Him, hearts rather than bodies would be circumcised, so that all who believe could become children of the covenant. As Scripture says, *No, a person is a Jew who is one inwardly; and circumcision is circumcision of the heart.*[cvii]

As we move ahead to the time of Moses, God gave Israel the covenant of the law, which placed a strong spotlight on the curse tied to the flesh. After giving the law, God required the Israelites to obey it in every detail, even though they were still living in fallen, sinful flesh. In effect, God laid out an impossible list of commands and then promised blessing for obedience and curses for failure.

In an earlier chapter, I discussed the wide range of fleshly curses listed in Deuteronomy 30 through 32. The law made it clear that sinful flesh leads to death, not only in an eternal sense, but also in everyday life.

Hundreds of years passed, and much of the Old Testament tells the story of Israel's repeated disobedience and the suffering that followed. They simply could not keep the law. In Romans 7, Paul explains that the law itself was not the problem. God's law was good and spiritual. The real issue was human flesh. All along, the law was meant to reveal the weakness of the flesh and the need for the curse of death to be brought to an end.

[cvi] Genesis 17:11 & 13
[cvii] Romans 2:29

For while we were living in the flesh, our sinful passions, aroused by the law, were at work in our members to bear fruit for death.

For we know that the law is spiritual, but I am of the flesh, sold under sin.

For since death came through a man, the resurrection of the dead comes also through a man. For as in Adam all die, so in Christ all will be made alive.[cviii]

There is one more part of the law given to Moses on Mount Sinai that points directly to the death of Jesus. A lesser-known command said that a body should not be left hanging overnight, because anyone who was hung on a pole was considered under God's curse. Later, in the New Testament, Paul refers back to this law when he explains what happened at the cross. *Christ redeemed us from the curse of the law by becoming a curse for us, for it is written: "Cursed is everyone who is hung on a pole."*[cix]

The Bread of Heaven

Until I began tracing the thread of the flesh throughout Scripture, I had no idea how far-reaching it really was. The significance of Christ's body, or His flesh, is enormous.

In a lesson that must have left many of His listeners confused, Jesus spoke about His body as the true bread from heaven. In that moment, He began to explain, in symbolic language, the very elements that would later take center stage in communion.

Then they asked him, "What must we do to do the works God requires?"

[cviii] Romans 7:5, 14, & 24-25
[cix] Galatians 3:13

Our ancestors ate the manna in the wilderness; as it is written: 'He gave them bread from heaven to eat.'"

Jesus said to them, "Very truly I tell you, it is not Moses who has given you the bread from heaven, but it is my Father who gives you the true bread from heaven.

I am the living bread that came down from heaven. If anyone eats of this bread, he will live forever. And the bread that I will give for the life of the world is my flesh...Truly, truly, I say to you, unless you eat the flesh of the Son of Man and drink his blood, you have no life in you. It is the Spirit who gives life; the flesh is no help at all. The words that I have spoken to you are spirit and life.[cx]

What did Jesus mean by all of this talk about eating His flesh? The people were simply asking what they needed to do to please God. They pointed back to the time in the wilderness when God gave their ancestors manna to eat, and Jesus responded, in a way that must have seemed puzzling, by saying that He Himself was the true bread from heaven.

The message He was giving through this metaphor[cxi] helps us understand the two great accomplishments of the cross.

So let us look back at the story in Numbers 11, where God provided manna, a truly unique bread from heaven. This bread was God's complete provision for His people. According to Jesus, it also pointed ahead to Himself, the true bread from heaven. Both manna and the Messiah required only faith and acceptance from those who wanted to receive their benefit. The Israelites had to trust that manna would

---

[cx] John 6:28, 31-32, 51, 53, & 63

[cxi] There are several ways we know this is a metaphor and not speaking of literally eating the body of Christ. Consider other metaphors speaking of Christ such as him being a door or a gate (Jn 10:9), a lamb (Jn 1:29), a shepherd (Heb 13:20), manna (Jn 6:23), light of the world (Jn 9:5), & the vine (Jn 15:1-5). Through these metaphors we gain insights into the nature and character of Jesus.

appear each day, which is why they were told to gather only enough for one day at a time. Both came from God, and both were entirely sufficient.

But the people wanted flesh! Although there are several Hebrew words that can mean meat, the word used in Numbers 11 is the same one used throughout the Old Testament for flesh. That specific word carries a symbolic connection to the curse, to death, and to the law. God became angry at their demands and, in essence, said, "You want flesh? I will give you so much flesh for a month that it will be coming out of your noses." [cxii]

Before I understood the spiritual meaning tied to the flesh, I thought God's strong reaction to their desire for a change in diet seemed excessive. Now it makes sense. Sin's curse on all flesh means that to walk in the flesh leads to death. The two go together. That is why it was fitting that a severe plague followed after God gave them the flesh they craved. God wanted to give them bread, which represented life, but they chose flesh, which represented death.

There are many more examples in Scripture that show this deep connection between physical flesh and the curse, but these are enough to highlight how important this theme is throughout the Bible.

Now let us return to the meaning God intended through both the flesh and the blood in Christ's work at the cross. Once this foundation is in place, the applications for health and healing begin to come into focus. So please bear with me as we take this next step together.

The Body and Blood of Christ

When I used to think about the cross, like most people, I focused almost entirely on the atoning blood of Christ. I never really noticed that Scripture gives just as much attention to His flesh as it does to His blood. Take a moment to look at a few of the many references for yourself, and you will see what I mean.

[cxii] Numbers 11:18-20

- *Since we have confidence to enter the holy places by the <u>blood</u> of Jesus, by the new and living way that he opened for us through the curtain, that is, through his <u>flesh.</u>*(Hebrews 10:19-20 ESV)

- *Is not the <u>cup</u> of thanksgiving for which we give thanks a participation in the <u>blood</u> of Christ? And is not the <u>bread</u> that we break a participation in the <u>body</u> of Christ?* (1 Corinthians 10:16 NIV)

- *But now in Christ Jesus you who once were far off have been brought near by the <u>blood</u> of Christ. For he himself is our peace, who has made us both one and has broken down in his <u>flesh</u> the dividing wall of hostility by abolishing the law of commandments expressed in ordinances, that he might create in himself one new man in place of the two, so making peace, and might reconcile us both to God in one <u>body</u> through the cross, thereby killing the hostility.* (Ephesians 2:13-16 ESV)

- *For in him all the fullness of God was pleased to dwell, and through him to reconcile to himself all things, whether on earth or in heaven, making peace by the <u>blood</u> of his cross. And you, who once were alienated and hostile in mind, doing evil deeds, he has now reconciled in his <u>body of flesh</u> by his death, in order to present you holy and blameless and above reproach before him.*(Colossians 1:19-22 ESV)

Adam's sin brought a curse that resulted in both physical and spiritual death for all flesh. Jesus' death addressed both of those problems for everyone who looks to His provision in faith. This is why we can praise God for both the body and the blood, the bread and the cup. It becomes clear, then, that the body of Christ, His flesh, represents something distinct from the blood. This leads us to one of the reasons for His long and agonizing death: sanctification.

Hebrews 10:10 tells us *we have been made holy through the sacrifice of the body of Jesus Christ once for all.* Then, just a few verses later, verse 14 adds that by that *sacrifice he has made perfect forever those who are being made holy.* In other words, our sanctification, being set apart for God, is both immediate and ongoing.

In John 17:19, Jesus prays to the Father, *For them I sanctify myself, that they too may be truly sanctified.* The morally perfect Christ clearly did not need to be purified from sin. So what did He mean? He set Himself apart for God's purpose and took on our sin so that, through His body, we too might be set apart for God.

In bringing *many sons to glory,* Jesus, *the captain of their salvation,* sanctified Himself.[cxiii] The Jewish people were looking for a conquering Messiah, so the suffering of Jesus became a stumbling block to them. Yet, as the founder of salvation, it was fitting that He would fully enter into the physical suffering of flesh under the curse in order to bring deliverance from it. Hebrews 2 speaks directly to this:

> *Jesus, crowned with glory and honor because of the suffering of death, so that by the grace of God he might taste death for everyone.*
>
> *For it was fitting that he, for whom and by whom all things exist, in bringing many sons to glory, should make the founder of their salvation perfect through suffering. For he who sanctifies and those who are sanctified all have one source.*
>
> *Since therefore the children share in flesh and blood, he himself likewise partook of the same things, that through death he might destroy the one who has the power of death, that is, the devil, and deliver all those who through fear of death were subject to lifelong slavery.*(Hebrews 2:9-11, 14-16)

> *How much more severely do you think someone deserves to be punished who has trampled the Son of God underfoot, who has treated as an unholy thing the blood of the covenant that sanctified them, and who has insulted the Spirit of grace? For we know him who said, "It is mine to avenge; I will repay," and*

[cxiii] Hebrews 2:11

again, "The Lord will judge his people." It is a dreadful thing to fall into the hands of the living God.

Jesus was a substitutionary sacrifice in more than one way, because He came to earth to address more than one problem. To resolve our separation from God, He shed His blood and took upon Himself the death that our sin demanded. To address the suffering that our sin brings, He willingly endured suffering in our place. As 1 Peter 1:24 says, *He himself bore our sins in his body on the cross, so that we might die to sins and live for righteousness; by his wounds you have been healed.*

Through the provision of both the body and the blood of Christ, those who believe in Him are no longer slaves to the desires of the flesh or to the death that comes from living according to the flesh.

With this understanding, we can see why taking communion with an unrepentant heart results in the Lord's discipline, which may come in the form of illness or even death. The many passages I have quoted show that Christ's suffering in His body at the cross is our provision for healing, and that this is inseparably connected to His blood, which was shed for the forgiveness of sin.

To show disrespect for the body and blood of Christ is to fail to examine one's own heart and truly turn away from sin. When that does not happen, God Himself brings judgment on the heart. According to 1 Corinthians 11:31–32, that judgment can take the form of illness and sometimes death. Hebrews 10:29–31 also speaks to the seriousness of showing contempt for the body of Christ.

The Two-Part Work of the Cross Seen in Passover

The biblical holiday most familiar to many Christians is probably Passover, which commemorates the events that led to Israel's exodus from slavery in Egypt. After nine devastating plagues, ranging from water turned to blood to storms of hail and swarms of frogs, God told Moses to prepare the people for a final act of judgment. This last plague would strike down every firstborn male in Egypt.

In Exodus 12, Moses gives the Israelites clear instructions so they might escape the death angel's mission. Each household was to slaughter a spotless lamb or goat and then do two very specific things with it. First, they were to place its blood on the sides and the top of their doorframe. Then they were to go inside and eat all the meat of the animal, along with unleavened bread and bitter herbs.

When this story is told, the focus usually stays on the blood placed on the doorposts and how it points to the blood Jesus shed so that we might be spared from God's wrath against sin. Yet the blood tells only half of the story. Eating the flesh, together with the bread and herbs, is just as deliberate and just as meaningful.

In Scripture, leaven, or yeast, often represents sin. That is why the Israelites were commanded to clear their homes of yeast during the week of Passover. The unleavened bread points forward to the body of Jesus, the true bread from heaven. The flesh of the lamb, eaten with bitter herbs, foreshadows the bitter suffering the Messiah would endure.

By eating the meal, the people were not only marking their homes for protection, they were also receiving, in a visible and tangible way, the provision God had made for their deliverance. In the same way that communion holds together both the body and the blood, Passover powerfully foreshadows the two-part work of Christ at the cross.

The Spirit Gives Life

I will close with one final and crucial piece of the puzzle, and it comes from the passage in Hebrews 10— *the Spirit of grace.* Remember, the Godhead works together as a perfect unit, with each Person fulfilling His role. Jesus, the spotless Lamb, made atonement for our sin, but it was the Holy Spirit who raised Him from the dead, making it possible for Him to conquer death. As Romans 8:11 reminds us, *He who raised Christ from the dead will also give life to your mortal bodies because of his Spirit who lives in you.*[cxiv]

[cxiv] Romans 8:11

It is by that same Spirit that we too are given life—not only eternally, but day by day. As we walk according to the Spirit, participating in ongoing sanctification, we receive the benefit of life, which includes healing. Many hope for a sudden, miraculous restoration—and sometimes it does happen. But whether healing comes quickly or gradually, it flows as a natural result of the sanctification of the flesh. The flesh always leads to death, but the Spirit always brings life.

As we journey through the wilderness of this life, the question becomes simple yet profound: will we, by faith, choose to feed daily on the Bread of Heaven, or will we turn to the desires of the flesh? The provision for healing here on this earth was accomplished at immense cost. If we want to experience that benefit, it is ours—but only when we receive it on God's terms.

Biblical Principle: *Jesus' suffering at the cross conquered the curse of the flesh (death), making provision through sanctification so that we can be healed.*

Call to Action: *Take some time to read all of Hebrews 10 in light of your understanding from this chapter. Worship the Lord with a thankful heart for all that He has accomplished for you.*

CHAPTER 13

Healing Today

For if you live according to the flesh you will die, but if by the Spirit you put to death the deeds of the body, you will live.
Romans 8:13

Menopause--a time in life hated and dreaded by women. Hormonal shifts that cause hot flashes, night sweats, the loss of any remaining metabolism, and moods that change as frequently as the weather in Iceland are just a few of the miseries that can characterize life for middle-aged women, often for years. To my dismay, my turn had come.

After more than eight years of good health, I found myself dealing with hormonal fluctuations that mystified and greatly interfered with any hope of looking at health from a merely academic perspective. Once again, I had the opportunity to test the biblical principles of health as my path of life headed into the swamps.

A Biblical Perspective of Health

Throughout this book, I have carefully laid out a biblical perspective on health and illness that often runs contrary to the assumption that health lies purely in the physical realm. The medical perspective presumes that symptoms originate with some part of the body breaking or malfunctioning. In recent decades, medicine has also considered an emotional component to illness, but, in their thinking, this lies solely in the physical realm and, therefore, is often treated chemically.

To use menopause as an example, most assume that the miseries that ensue come purely from hormonal imbalances as the body transitions. They can run tests to determine what those precise hormone levels are and then boost those levels synthetically or naturally. Attempting to manipulate the body manually has its issues though, not just with menopause but with all illnesses, as the treatment often creates new symptoms or illnesses. This purely physical approach to health through testing, drugs, surgery, physical therapy, diet, exercise, or the like seems to make sense and to do or think otherwise appears foolish and perhaps even dangerous.

Although something malfunctioning in the body will certainly produce symptoms, the actual cause of the malfunction likely has little to do with the body itself. The biblical perspective of health reveals a direct connection between the physical and the spiritual. Chronic illness persists when the two are in conflict. Therefore, healing begins with determining why the physical is being negatively influenced by the spiritual. Romans 8:13 summarizes the matter by saying, *For if you live according to the flesh you will die, but if by the Spirit you put to death the deeds of the body, you will live.*

When Christians pray for healing, it is generally with hope for miracles along the lines of the New Testament examples. The problem with that expectation is that the dramatic and miraculous healings of the Gospels and Acts occurred because of God's grace as He demonstrated the power and authority of the Son of God and the apostles so that the Gospel might be spread throughout the world.[cxv] Other than that, the Bible primarily describes miracles being performed by people and at

---

[cxv] 1 Thessalonians 1:5 *our gospel came to you not simply with words but also with power*

times when God was doing something unique, such as with Moses and the prophets.

However, one pattern has remained constant--that of the flesh bringing death and the Spirit bringing life and peace. That thread runs throughout all of time as Genesis to Revelation reveals. Under the covenant of the law, God highlighted the weakness of the flesh and the results of living according to its desires. He gave the sacrifices as a means to avoid the wrath disobedience incurred. In the church age, the apostles healed as Jesus did but taught that the path of life is through the sanctification of the Spirit. The need for sacrifices no longer exists because Jesus' sacrifice made provision for atonement and life once and for all. Not that miracles do not still occur, but the provision for healing, miraculous or otherwise, comes through the sanctification of the flesh.

Set Free from the Law of Sin & Death

During the time of writing the last chapter on how Jesus conquered the curse of the flesh, I went out for my daily walk and prayer time. The August heat and oppressive humidity that met me as I stepped out the front door did nothing for my hormonal state of mind and body. As I walked, thoughts and concerns of the abdominal pain that years ago characterized my days and had recently returned called for my attention. A heart-to-heart talk with my loving Savior was needed, and the familiar paths I traversed provided a fitting venue.

As I laid out to the Lord my litany of complaints, concerns, and questions, the content of the Scriptures that I had been studying came to mind. The Holy Spirit directed my thoughts to the familiar words of one of my favorite chapters in the Bible--Romans 8. *For the law of the Spirit of life has set you free in Christ Jesus from the law of sin and death.*[cxvi] Sin AND death. There it was again--the two problems dealt

---

[cxvi] Romans 8:2 (This verse and the coming verses from Romans 8 are from the ESV.)

with through the cross. Because Jesus suffered and died on the cross, He atoned for our sin and conquered death (the curse of the flesh).

Watchman Nee, the author of <u>The Normal Christian Life</u>, uses the illustration of gravity to illustrate how the law of the Spirit of Life overcomes the law of sin and death. The law of gravity dictates that if something falls, it will be pulled downward. However, the law of gravity can be overcome. If an apple falls but I catch it, I have overcome the law of gravity so that the normal course of the law is arrested. By my power, a greater force, the apple does not fall to the ground.

No thanks to Adam and Eve, the law of sin and death became a relentless reality for all mankind, and all became slaves to that law. People needed a greater force to overcome the law of sin and death for them. And so, Romans 8 goes on to explain how Jesus accomplished this:

For God has done what the law, weakened by the flesh, could not do. By sending his own Son in the likeness of sinful flesh and for sin, he condemned sin in the flesh, in order that the righteous requirement of the law might be fulfilled in us... (vs.3-4)

A greater power, God Himself, overcame the certainty of the law that once ruled the flesh--sin and death. Although salvation depends on understanding and believing that the Son of God, in the flesh, accomplished these things for us, the reality of just how that applies to daily life escapes most.

As I walked and talked with the Lord, I found myself making excuses for my moods, irritableness, complaining, and gloomy thoughts. I knew that my heart was not at peace and that I now frequently walked according to the flesh. Nothing big, mind you, but my fuse had grown rather short. Surely, I was a victim of my circumstances (the shifting hormonal balance); therefore, it could not be held against me. I was helpless. I did not ask to go through this. As Americans love to say these days, "It is what it is." Right? But God's

answer for what seemed to be my legitimate argument came in the
verses that follow as Romans 8 continues.

> *who walk not according to the flesh but according to the Spirit.*
> *For those who live according to the flesh set their minds on the*
> *things of the flesh, but those who live according to the Spirit set*
> *their minds on the things of the Spirit. For to set the mind on the*
> *flesh is death, but to set the mind on the Spirit is life and peace.*
> *For the mind that is set on the flesh is hostile to God, for it does*
> *not submit to God's law; indeed, it cannot. Those who are in the*
> *flesh cannot please God.* (vs.4-8)

I recognized that I frequently had my mind focused on matters
of the flesh--how I felt, worries about what my body was doing,
complaints about anything or anyone who made my issues more of a
burden, and so on. This focus on the needs and demands of the flesh
seemed appropriate and inescapable, but they stole my peace and were
sin. The thought occurred to me, "I wonder if I repented and allowed
my focus to be on the things of the Spirit, if my hormonal symptoms
might subside?" The time had come to put the following biblical
principle to the test: **To walk according to the flesh brings death but
to walk according to the Spirit brings life and peace.**

Going back to the illustration of the law of gravity, let me
substitute a baby for the apple. All those who have ever held a baby
know that they are prone to squirm. Their natural inclination to
constantly move about and their lack of understanding of the
consequences of the law of gravity makes them likely to wiggle right
out of the safe arms of the one holding them. Every noise, light, or
shifting shadow grabs their focus, and they attempt to move in curious
response.

Because of the resurrection power of the Spirit of life living in us,
we have overcome the law of sin and death. The Lord holds us fast, and
while abiding in Him, we reap the benefit of the Spirit (life and peace).
We could, however, like a wiggling baby, fall prey to the effects of

natural law at any moment. The former law, after all, remains, and we become subject to its effects (sin and death) every time we choose to exit the grasp of the One who has overcome that law for us.

Excuses

What occurred to me as I walked and talked with the Lord that day was that the circumstances of the flesh will always be present and screaming for my attention. For now, the move towards menopause provides me with a noisy distraction from the things of the Spirit, but if it was not that, something else would take its place. As humans, we constantly have the physical, mental, and emotional responses of the flesh attracting our attention, especially in difficult circumstances. Satan loves to use those distractions to bring us back into captivity. But we are no longer slaves to the flesh because Jesus has overcome the curse of the flesh, and the Spirit dwells in us.

Think about your own circumstances. Are you in a high stress job or perhaps caring for a child with special needs? Is your marriage falling apart? Do you have an illness that causes debilitating pain or other symptoms? Are you a young mom whose children consume your energy and push you to your limit day after day? Do you deal with depression or anxiety? Whatever your struggles, do you feel like a slave to them and your inability to rise above their effects a foregone conclusion? Do you find yourself disregarding or even excusing your sinful thoughts, attitudes, and actions with the thought that until the current circumstances come to an end, this is how you will be? "It is what it is!"

The truth for the Christian, though, is that we are no longer slaves to the flesh. Stop and think about that truth. Satan would have you believe that your circumstances will dictate your behavior, but that is a lie from the pit of hell.

Christ overcame for us so that we might have the Spirit's resurrection power to walk in new life. It is in the process of the Spirit's sanctifying work that we learn to keep our focus on the things of the Spirit, rather than the things of the flesh. When the flesh screams for our attention, we can respond as Jesus did when He too agonized in the weakness of the flesh in the garden. Three times He wrestled in prayer that He might focus on thoughts of the Father's will rather than His own.

Ten days have now passed since I repented of walking according to the flesh and instead began to follow the instruction of 2 Corinthians 10:5. *We demolish arguments and every pretension that sets itself up against the knowledge of God, and we take captive every thought to make it obedient to Christ.* I am thrilled with the outcome! My hormonal symptoms, including moods, tiredness, and abdominal pain have ceased. I have even lost a couple of pounds without changing the way I eat. Honestly, I am energized! The almost immediate response of my body to the truth of Romans 8:6 astounds me-- *The mind governed by the flesh is death, but the mind governed by the Spirit is life and peace.*

Pain Illustrates the Power of the Mind

The way the body perceives pain illustrates, in the physical realm, the spiritual truth of Romans 8. In Norman Doidge, M.D.'s second book, The Brain's Way of Healing, he explains the significant change in the way science now understands the body's pain response. The "common sense" thinking about pain that persists today but has now been proven completely wrong, came from Rene Descartes' theory four hundred years ago. I imagine you will recognize his ideas. His theory said,

> *when we are hurt, our pain nerves send a one-way signal up to the brain, and the intensity of the pain is proportional to the seriousness of our injury. In other words, pain files an accurate damage report about the extent of the body's injury, and that the role of the brain is to simply accept that report.*[54]

In 1965 two neuroscientists, Ronald Melzak and Patrick Wall overturned Descartes' theory of pain with the "gate control theory of pain."[55] This, now accepted but vastly different theory teaches that the brain itself controls how much pain we feel. Injured tissue relays messages that must pass through "gates" or controls beginning in the spinal cord and continuing to the brain. These messages can only proceed to the brain if the brain gives "permission" for the various gates to open. If a gate is opened, the feeling of pain increases *by allowing certain neurons to turn on and transmit their signals*"[56] If the brain does not open the gate, then it blocks the *pain signal by releasing endorphins, the narcotics made by our bodies to quell pain.*[57]

Doidge tells how world-renowned pain specialist and psychiatrist, Michael Moskowitz, MD had the misfortune of personally testing the gate theory of pain when he fell and completely broke the longest bone in his body, the femur. With his leg jutting out at a 90-degree angle from itself, the pain he felt was a true ten out of ten. However, as he waited for the ambulance, he discovered that within about sixty seconds of his lying completely still, the pain vanished. Because the brain uses pain as a means of protecting the body from further injury, once Moskowitz stopped moving, the brain perceived that the threat of harm to his leg had ended, and so it closed the gate, so to speak, on the pain messages. When the paramedics arrived and moved him, his pain immediately returned to a ten.

As a pain specialist doctor, Moskowitz knowledgeably ordered the paramedics to give him a higher than typical dose of morphine to avoid the likelihood that his acute (short-lived) pain might later turn into a chronic pain condition. By limiting the frequency of pain signals through morphine, he could possibly avoid lasting changes to his brain. He knew that, as I described in chapter seven, the brain's plasticity allows changes to be made to itself as a result of neurons repeatedly firing in response to a specific trigger (neurons that wire together fire together).

Furthermore, science now understands that as pain signals continue day after day, they cause the plastic brain to ever-encroach on nearby areas of the brain producing an increasingly wider and more intense degree of pain.[58] Because the pain actually exists in the brain and not in the injury itself, chronic pain signals, in a sense, lie to us as they spread their associations to more and more parts of the body.

Let us consider Romans 8:6 in light of the illustration of pain. *The mind governed by the flesh is death, but the mind governed by the Spirit is life and peace.* Our flesh, ruled by the sin-nature, sends continual messages, similar to pain signals, in an attempt to get us to take notice so that we might feed the desires of the soul. The messages spring from endless triggers. These thoughts must then pass through the gates of our spirit. If our spirit allows the Holy Spirit to shut the gate on the sinful desires, then the physical effects of the curse of sin and death are replaced with life and peace.

Similar to when the brain stops neural messages of pain at the gates and sends back endorphins in their place, the mind of the Spirit must counter the desires of the flesh to breathe life into our mortal bodies. When we take every thought captive and replace them with God's truth, then we allow the Holy Spirit to be the gatekeeper of our minds. What is the mind of God? Philippians 4:8 says, *Whatever is true, whatever is noble, whatever is right, whatever is pure, whatever is lovely, whatever is admirable—if anything is excellent or praiseworthy—think about such things.*

Take Action

I realized that, if my mind was to be governed by the Spirit, merely stopping the messages stemming from the menopausal condition of my body with Scripture at a given moment was second best. Preventing that battle in the first place by allowing the mind of the Spirit to govern at all times would work far better.

Think about how the brain ended all of Moskowitz' pain once his movement stopped. Merely continuing to hold still and feel no pain was much easier than having to fight the intense urge to writhe for sixty seconds while pain messages screamed at him; "Move! It hurts!" The same proves true in benefiting from the Spirit's life and peace. Constantly fighting individual battles to go against the cravings of the flesh is much harder than following Paul's counsel in Romans 13:14. *But put on the Lord Jesus Christ, and make no provision for the flesh, to gratify its desires.* Once the "provision" has been made, the battle begins.

I began to think through and ask the Lord to show me how I was making provision for the flesh. He brought a number of things to mind. Complaining was one. Just think about what is required in order to complain: One must focus on the desires of the flesh! Grumbling coming out of the mouth indicates the mind is focused on the desires of the flesh, not on the mind of the Spirit. *Make no provision for the flesh.* Complaining became to me a warning light, alerting me to my unhealthy focus.

Another change I made was to choose more carefully what I set my mind on in entertainment. There may not be anything wrong with relaxing by watching television or enjoying many other forms of entertainment, but it does powerfully feed the flesh. Even if it happens to be "clean," the topics covered and the lifestyle, attitudes, or ways of thinking portrayed, more often than not, encourage fleshly thoughts that are not good and praiseworthy. I needed to limit this input significantly to keep my mind governed by the Spirit.

A third area that I needed to improve on was to prevent my thoughts from turning to a fleshly focus in the first place by singing more worship songs of praise and praying. Doing so at times when I know I am prone to negative thoughts is especially important. To do so clothed me with Christ. If Paul and Silas could sing praises in prison, then I could sing praises as I work about the house.[cxvii]

The areas you struggle with the flesh might be different than mine. I encourage you to think about where you make provision for the flesh, to gratify its desires. Then, do not merely determine to fight those

---

[cxvii] Acts 16:25

battles with sin's temptation, but to avoid the battle in the first place by clothing yourself with the mind of the Spirit throughout your day.

The Realm of the Spirit

As I have contemplated the biblical principle that the flesh brings death, but the Spirit gives life and peace, I have wondered how this is? The answer ties together all the biblical principles of health. The curse on all flesh produces constant deterioration, day after day, leading eventually to its death, both on this earth and then for eternity. To feed the flesh is to give the curse full reign.

For the spiritually lost, their health can greatly benefit simply through mind-over-mater disciplines (positive thinking and the like) and right living. Science bears out the impact of the heart giving life to the body and the benefits of right living, i.e., moderation in consumption of food and drink, avoiding illicit sex, etc. However, as demonstrated by the Israelites under the law, overcoming the cravings of the flesh through willpower alone proves unsustainable at best.

For the saved, the law of sin and death remains in place, but we are not slaves to it, thanks to the immediate and on-going sanctification of the Spirit. Romans 8 continues to elaborate on this truth by saying,

You, however, are not in the realm of the flesh but are in the realm of the Spirit, if indeed the Spirit of God lives in you. And if anyone does not have the Spirit of Christ, they do not belong to Christ. But if Christ is in you, then even though your body is subject to death because of sin, the Spirit gives life because of righteousness. And if the Spirit of him who raised Jesus from the dead is living in you, he who raised Christ from the dead will also give life to your mortal bodies because of his Spirit who lives in you.[cxviii]

[cxviii] Romans 8:9-11

So, through the Spirit, two things happen that greatly benefit our health. First, we have the power to walk in peace, an emotional state that causes the body to function as God designed it to best function. Second, we have life breathed into our bodies by the Giver of Life. In these ways, the mind governed by the Spirit has life and the relentless physical effects of the curse are arrested. These benefits of life to the body are provided for all of God's children.

The downside, however, for a child of God is that the Father often disciplines those who persist in walking according to the flesh by specifically targeting the flesh through illness.[cxix] The upside, however, is that the Father desperately loves His children and desires to bring healing if they will only repent and walk again according to the Spirit.

This healing may be immediate and miraculous but more often comes gradually as we continue to walk in righteousness. In the Bible, healing occurred through a variety of methods such as words, mud, a poultice of figs, water, and touch, just to name a few. Healing also occurred in different time frames, sometimes immediately, sometimes with a delay, and sometimes over time. The healing of today as a part of sanctification varies just as widely as in biblical times. God will faithfully heal as His children walk in righteousness, but He alone chooses what that healing will look like.

I often receive questions from people who deal with chronic illness. Some acknowledge their need for repentance, as well as pursuing a knowledge of God rather than endlessly pursuing doctors, tests, and the like. The question then arises, "But what do I do about...?"(fill in the blank with the symptom). "Should I stop taking my supplements? Should I eat this or not eat that?" Such questions are natural, and I, unfortunately, do not have the answers. God alone holds that knowledge. I only know that when God's children allow their minds to be governed by the Spirit, they will have life. Pray and ask for wisdom and direction to know the means that the Lord would

---

[cxix] 1 Corinthians 10: 5-11 & 11:30-32

choose to bring healing to you. Rest in Him and let the Spirit do what He does best--give life.

I shared in the last chapter, the story of the Israelites craving meat (flesh) in the wilderness rather than manna. If you recall, according to Jesus those events picture how God's children should feed on Him, the bread of Heaven, not on the flesh. With the eating of the flesh came death. Sin and death always go together. Do you want to be well? Do you pray and long for complete healing? Then eat of the Bread of Heaven, not of the flesh. Jesus made the provision through His body on a tree. He has overcome the law of sin and death and in Him, you have new life. Walk in it.

So then, brothers, we are debtors, not to the flesh, to live according to the flesh. For if you live according to the flesh you will die, but if by the Spirit you put to death the deeds of the body, you will live.[cxx]

Biblical Principle: *To walk according to the flesh brings death but to walk according to the Spirit brings life and peace.*

Call to Action: *Consider where you "make provision for the flesh, to gratify its desires." Think through and ask the Lord to help you to determine changes that should occur in your daily life to allow your mind to be governed by the Spirit rather than the flesh.*

[cxx] Romans 8:12-13

CHAPTER 14

Not All Illness Is Spiritual

"Rabbi, who sinned, this man or his parents, that he was born blind?" "Neither this man nor his parents sinned," said Jesus.
John 9:2-3

I remember watching the unfolding of a scene in the movie *Miracles From Heaven*, based on the true story of the Beam family whose young daughter, Anna, developed a rare disease that left her unable to digest food.[59] In this particular scene, the Beam family attends their church one Sunday morning during the early days of their child's horrific illness. Following the service, friends of the deeply struggling mother, Christy Beam, approach her.

Under the circumstances, one might expect the friends to offer hugs and words of comfort with promises to pray. Instead, with conspiratorial glances, the spokeswoman of the group informs Christy that she needs to pray about what sin she might have committed that led God to punish her child through sickness. My heart broke for the pain those "friends" caused this poor mother in her hour of great need. Even if those ladies had the best of intentions, their approach proved devastating, driving Christy from the doors of the church and from the Lord she desperately needed.

Lest anyone misconstrue the message and intent of the last several chapters, I must emphatically state the next biblical principle. **Not every illness is the result of personal sin or the absence of peace.** In fact, the Bible gives two extremely clear cases, one in each Testament, as well as other explanations for disease that serve to caution one from dogmatically connecting every sickness to a lack of peace with God, oneself, or others.

While the preponderance of Scripture indicates that much illness stems from a lack of peace, often due to sin, the awareness of other causes should bring significant pause to those inclined to judge people who are sick. Throughout the ages, the church has often caused much anguish to hurting people. Let us take caution, then, to avoid perpetuating that record of harm.

Old Testament Example --Job

The book of Job provides a detailed and explicit example of the fact that not all illness indicates a heart issue. Chapter 1 gives us a rare, inside look into the events of the spirit realm. Satan asks permission of God to test Job's devotion to the Lord with a dreadful assault on every area of the righteous man's life. In four waves, Job learns of the loss of all of his property, including servants and livestock, and the deaths of every one of his ten children. The author tells us of Job's worshipful response to the Giver and Taker of Life, in spite of such overwhelming devastation, and concludes the chapter with, *In all this, Job did not sin by charging God with wrongdoing* (1:22).

Chapter 2 begins with another inside look. In a follow-up conversation between God and Satan, the Almighty grants permission for the Evil One to physically harm Job, as long as his life is spared. As a result, Satan afflicts Job with a nightmarish case of boils that covers him from the *soles of his feet to the top of his head* (2:7).

At this point, an utterly broken Job collapses in dust and ashes while scraping his sores with broken pottery. Despite an unimaginable level of misery and devastation, Job does not sin. Repeatedly, the text makes clear that the cause of the illness resulting in boils is not because of any fault with Job. In fact, the exact opposite is true. He lived so righteously, and God blessed him so abundantly that Satan took notice.

Desiring to help, Job's "friends" come to offer their comfort and advice. As people tend to do, Job's friends saw his pitiful state and determined to help him fix the situation. Their exhortations centered on a firm belief that, to have warranted such an onslaught of suffering, Job must have had some area of sin in his life. Despite Job's declarations of innocence, in long speeches, they repeatedly insisted that he should repent of whatever sin he had committed so that he might obtain mercy from God. Talk about beating someone when he is down!

In the end, God silenced the men and spoke directly to Job. Never once, however, did the Almighty give Job an explanation for his suffering. Only we hold that insight. However, God did openly rebuke the other men for their incorrect assessment of Job's situation and required them to go to Job, who then offered sacrifices for their sins against him and prayed for them. The book ends with the report that God blessed Job greater in the second half of his life than in the first.

New Testament Example--The Blind Man

Another clear indication that not all illness is the result of God's discipline for sin is the story of Jesus healing the man born blind found in John chapter 9. In this account, the disciples ask Jesus about the man they encounter. *"Rabbi, who sinned, this man or his parents, that he was born blind?" "Neither this man nor his parents sinned,"* said Jesus, *"but this happened so that the works of God might be displayed in him* (John 9:2-3). In other words, the man was blind for the very purpose that his healing might bring glory to God. Now, that is an interesting thought!

It would appear that God had the same purpose in mind for young Anna Beam. Yes, she suffered tremendously from the effects of her "incurable" illness for quite some time. However, at the time God sovereignly established, He miraculously healed her. How? While climbing a dead tree, the child fell into its hollow center and remained unconscious throughout a prolonged rescue effort to remove her. When she emerged, God had fully restored little Anna to health. Her story, as written by her mother, has now become a major motion picture that credits God with her impossible healing.

As stories like those of Anna and the blind man reveal, we must not presume, in our limited knowledge, to know why a particular illness has occurred. Neither do we know how God intends to work through that illness.

Note, however, that the disciples' question to Jesus about whether the man or his parents had sinned expressed the common assumption by the Jews that all illness stemmed from sin. Where did they get such an idea? They did not just pull the question out of thin air! The law of Moses and the covenant of the Old Testament emphatically stated that God disciplines His children for sin in multiple ways, but especially through illness. Furthermore, the disciples had heard Jesus frequently say, upon healing someone, "your sins are forgiven."

In fact, on one occasion, after healing an invalid of thirty-eight years, Jesus said to the man, *See, you are well again. Stop sinning or something worse may happen to you.*[cxxi]   Clearly, then, the Son of God frequently connected illness with sin. In spite of this, Jesus' response to the disciples after the healing of the blind man specifically demonstrates that sin is not the root of every illness or infirmity. We must not forget this!

Illness Associated With Old Age

In addition to the reasons evidenced in the book of Job and in the ninth chapter of John, a biblical case can be made for other sources of illness unrelated to spiritual well-being. One is illness associated with old age. Another is illness due to the fact that we live in a fallen world.

[cxxi] John 5:14

While the Bible tells that God does occasionally bring a peaceful death to His elderly servants without a decline in health, strength, and vitality, (Moses for example[cxxii]), the general rule experienced by the majority is that health declines with age. Most often, God allows the normal process of aging to take its course, as with Isaac, Jacob, and David.

In Ecclesiastes twelve, Solomon offers a poetic description of the physical effects of old age. He speaks of weakness and trembling, the loss of hearing, sight, teeth, and sexual desire, and eventually death. Such age-related degeneration originates in the fall of Adam and Eve. Solomon writes:

> *Remember your Creator in the days of your youth, before the days of trouble come...when the keepers of the house tremble, and the strong men stoop, when the grinders cease because they are few, and those looking through the windows grow dim; when...the sound of grinding fades; when men rise up at the sound of birds, but all their songs grow faint...the grasshopper drags himself along and desire no longer is stirred. Then man goes to his eternal home.[cxxiii]*

The Bible also says in Psalm 90:10, *The years of our life are seventy, or even by reason of strength eighty; yet their span is but toil and trouble; they are soon gone, and we fly away* (ESV). Modern medicine might prolong the span of life, but as this verse states, the years will be full of toil and trouble. That toil may or may not have anything to do with God's discipline.

Because of what I see in Scripture, my recommendation for anyone over seventy who struggles with their health would initially be the same as that for any young person: Pray that God might reveal any areas of sin or areas lacking peace. If needed, repent and ask for healing. If the Holy Spirit does not reveal sin or the absence of peace,

---

[cxxii] Deuteronomy 34:5-7
[cxxiii] Ecclesiastes 12:1-5

then someone over seventy might pray for healing but then rest in the eternal hope promised for all those who have salvation. Paul's words and perspective in 2 Timothy 4:6-8 provide excellent encouragement in such cases.

> *For I am already being poured out like a drink offering, and the time for my departure is near. I have fought the good fight, I have finished the race, I have kept the faith. Now there is in store for me the crown of righteousness, which the Lord, the righteous Judge, will award to me on that day—and not only to me, but also to all who have longed for his appearing.*

Illness Due to a Fallen World

We know from Galatians 4:13 that God used illness to bring Paul to the Galatians that he might preach the Gospel to people who were ready to receive it. Although nowhere does it state whether his illness was or was not the result of sin, we know that God brought great good out of it. Because we live in a fallen world, illnesses from bacteria, viruses, and general degeneration make up our existence. Most likely, Paul's illness, in this case, stemmed from such a cause.

Similarly, an episode with the flu, for example, most likely has nothing to do with the sin of the sick individual. After all, the Genesis curse affects the righteous and the unrighteous. A sovereign God could choose, however, to use a germ for discipline just as easily as He used a germ to place Paul in the right situation for sharing the Gospel. Although it never hurts to search your heart for unrepented sin, in cases of short-lived illnesses that are common to man, do not let fear and condemnation rule your heart. However, if the initial illness becomes chronic (prolonged), then take special notice.

In all cases, never forget the biblical principle that a heart at peace gives life to the body. When the heart is in turmoil, the body's ability to heal and revive itself diminishes greatly.

Speaking the Truth in Love

The clear examples from Job and the healing of the blind man firmly establish that **not every illness is the result of personal sin or the absence of peace**. Those examples, therefore, should serve as a strong hand of caution regarding how we address those who suffer from illness. Great sensitivity and love, along with an assumption of innocence should direct our encouragements and exhortations to those who are ill. We do not know another's heart, and we certainly cannot presume to know the way of God in a particular situation.

With that said, however, I want to pose a question. Is it loving to hide or ignore the biblical teachings that indicate an illness MIGHT be the result of a lack of peace in one's heart, or perhaps even that it is a result of God's loving discipline intended to bring an individual back into right fellowship with Him? Oh, how I wish I had known the truth years earlier!

When my courageous and loving friend gave me the "gift" of a book and shared with me her concerns that sin might be playing into my poor health, she followed the counsel of James 5. It says,

> *My brothers and sisters, if one of you should wander from the truth and someone should bring that person back, remember this: Whoever turns a sinner from the error of their way will save them from death and cover over a multitude of sins.*[cxxiv]

When God prompts us, we should gently speak the truth in love. If you feel called to speak of these matters to someone suffering from illness, I urge you to first spend an extended time in prayer. Ask the Lord to search your own heart so that you do not become guilty of trying to remove a speck from your neighbor's eye while a plank protrudes from your own (Matthew 7:3-5). Also, pray that God might heal your friend or loved one in spirit, soul, and body and prepare his/her heart for what you will share.

[cxxiv] James 5:19-20

If, after a time of prayer, you still believe God would have you raise your concerns to one who is ill, I strongly caution you against bringing up such matters in writing. The likelihood of causing offense increases exponentially when the individual cannot hear the love in your voice or have the opportunity to discuss or clarify when needed. You might also consider beginning with a humble, personal testimony or by first acknowledging the example of Job.

Finally, following your gentle prelude, consider simply giving them two or three Bible references written down on a piece of paper and ask your friend to read them and pray about whether or not they might apply. This allows God's Word and the Holy Spirit to do the speaking. Then, the loving Father who knows all will bring His good purposes to pass in His perfect time.

Biblical Principle: *Not every illness is the result of personal sin or the absence of peace.*

Call to Action: *Continue to seek God's personal revelation for any areas needing repentance, but if the Holy Spirit does not reveal anything of concern, choose to rest in your Savior's daily strength and provision for each day until His healing comes.*

Part 3

The Path of Life

CHAPTER 15

Self-Esteem or Christ-Esteem Finding True Inner Peace

For whenever our heart condemns us, God is greater than our heart, and he knows everything. 1 John 3:20 ESV

At seven years of age, when I still wore bows in my hair and skipped about as young children do, my world changed. In the woods that I loved to play in behind my house, I lost my innocence. For almost a year, the abuse continued, but I had no mental framework by which to interpret or understand those events. Then, at age eight, I spent the night with a friend who, with many nervous giggles, showed me a children's book on "the birds and the bees." With absolute horror, I realized I had lost something precious and irreplaceable. The conclusion drawn that night would reverberate in my mind for many years to come: "I was bad. No one will want me."

Like a fountain breaking forth from the deep, evidence of my inner turmoil surfaced. By day, I regularly helped myself to the Pepto Bismol in the bathroom to combat the frequent stomach aches that began to plague me. By night, my subconscious continued its torments through endless nightmares. As the second tallest child in my third-grade class at school, I found myself strangely compelled to beat up the boys during recess, and quite capable of doing so. No conscious reason existed for my actions, but anger at boys drove me.

By thirteen, self-accusations, confirmed by the rejection of others, convinced me of my unworthiness for love. Oh, how I longed to die. Anguish over the abuse continued through my teen years until, while a freshman in college, the Lord provided a lay counselor to lovingly guide me to emotional healing and a right understanding of the events of my childhood.

Although your story may be different from mine, chances are good that you too have known the torment of self-incrimination and guilt. Perhaps that condemnation still rings in your mind today. If so, regardless of whether such thoughts are the result of your own actions or those of another, one thing is certain: Lack of peace with yourself will greatly impact your health.

The wise King Solomon spoke of this in Proverbs 18:24: *The human spirit can endure in sickness, but a crushed spirit who can bear?* Is your heart broken? Do you carry burdens of guilt? Do you, on the whole, view yourself negatively, always falling short when you compare yourself to others? Might you even characterize your feelings toward yourself as hatred? Are you overly concerned with personal perfection and berate yourself mercilessly when you fail to meet those standards? If any of these ring true, the time has come to allow the loving Savior to bind up your broken heart so that it might begin to breathe life into every cell of your body.[cxxv]

In an earlier chapter, I mentioned the two greatest commandments found in Matthew 22:37-39. Within those commands, which summarize the entire law, we find the three, primary relationships where love is required--with God, with others, and with ourselves. It says, *Love the Lord your God with all your heart and with all your soul and with all your mind. This is the first and greatest commandment. And the second is like it: Love your neighbor as*

[cxxv] Proverbs 14:30

yourself. If we are to love our neighbors as ourselves, the assumption is that we must first love ourselves.

The Fragility of Self-Esteem

In the last couple of decades, teaching on self-esteem has flooded classrooms, little league sports, books on parenting, and homes throughout Europe and America. From such an abundance of "wisdom" and the widespread attempts at living accordingly, one might expect the current generation to be more at peace with themselves than any of those previous. Tragically, no.

2015 statistics, released by the National Health Services (a UK health organization), reported that the number of girls under eighteen in the UK who needed hospital treatment after poisoning themselves rose 42% in the last decade.[60] Furthermore, the number of girls requiring inpatient treatment for cutting themselves almost quadrupled over the same period--a 285% rise. Additionally, the girls who received treatment after hanging themselves also more than quadrupled.

Although the number for boys falls significantly below that of girls, the incidences of self-mutilation and hanging for boys also dramatically increased in the same ten-year period (a rise of 186% for hospital visits related to self-cutting and a 50% increase in hanging). Keep in mind that these numbers include only the incidences of teenage self-harm that resulted in hospital care, and therefore, provide only a glimpse into the magnitude of the total problem.

Although many theorize about the blame for this generation's despair, I draw this conclusion: The world's approach to building self-esteem fails to combat personal anguish. *Meriam Webster's Dictionary* defines self-esteem as "a confidence and satisfaction in oneself." We all desperately need this confidence and satisfaction; however, *Psychology Today* points out significant problems that arise from either too much or too little self-esteem.

Possessing little self-regard can lead people to become depressed, to fall short of their potential, or to tolerate abusive situations and relationships. Too much self-love, on the other hand, results in an off-putting sense of entitlement and an inability to learn from failures. (It can also be a sign of clinical narcissism.)[61]

Consider for a moment the subjective nature of self-esteem. When we personally evaluate our worth, we mentally hold up our good attributes against our bad to determine which outweighs the other. We also consider our successes and accomplishments against our failures. Throw in the fact that the way we evaluate those factors varies from day-to-day with our moods, as do the standards or people by which we compare ourselves. Additionally, negative voices from the past can echo endlessly and impact our present perception of personal worth.

Therefore, maintaining balanced self-esteem becomes a bit like walking a tightrope. Few can adjust to the constant shifts without falling to the side of too little or too much self-regard. Unfortunately, when this kind of inner conflict rules the heart, it negatively affects our health.

Christ-Esteem

How then can a right and unchanging sense of personal worth be achieved? Through truth! "But wait," you say. "I'm fat, unattractive, not smart enough, moody, not good with people, neurotic, or _____ (you fill in the blank), and that IS the truth!" However, all such self-judgments are based on changeable and subjective opinions. We need worth based on TRUTH.

Truth never changes or shifts because it lies solely in the person of Jesus Christ who is the Alpha and the Omega (the beginning and the end). He is ***the way and the truth and the life***.[cxxvi] When you know and

---

[cxxvi] John 14:6

abide in the Truth, you can be set free from many things[cxxvii]--including an ever-changing view of yourself based on personal assessment or the opinions of others. Christ-esteem, not self-esteem is needed to be at peace with oneself.

The One who fashioned you in His image and calls you by name also knows your every flaw and failure and still cherishes you. We know God takes into account our limitations because Psalm 103:14 says, *For he knows how we are formed. He remembers that we are dust.* Unbound by time and human limitations, the Almighty sees what you can be IN CHRIST.

Think of it this way--God sees you through the lens of Truth (Christ). His righteousness is yours! The resurrection He attained made it possible for you to be a new creation IN CHRIST! This is the truth of Christ-esteem and leads us to our next biblical principle of health: **Peace with myself comes from believing God's truth about me and brings health to my whole body.**

In Christ

I would like to take you back to the first phase of the ceremony of cleansing from infectious diseases discussed in chapter eight. In it, the priest declared the cleansed leper clean seven times (the number of completion). However, before such blessed words found utterance, the priest symbolically and prophetically demonstrated the complete picture of Jesus' work at the cross and the salvation that work made possible. Because of the Gospel, an individual is made worthy. THEN, the priest affirmed, "you are clean."

You might wonder why I draw attention to the order of these events. It is because, through this, we learn two simple yet critical truths. First, Christ alone makes a person worthy. Second, it is only because of Christ that God declares all who trust in Him clean. Those

---

[cxxvii] John 8:31-32 *To the Jews who had believed him, Jesus said, "If you hold to my teaching, you are really my disciples. Then you will know the truth, and the truth will set you free."*

two truths address the need of every heart to feel worthy (valuable, significant, and loved) and free from guilt and shame (cleansed). So often, though, people seek to meet these needs within themselves, rather than in Christ. Doing so makes inner peace quite fragile.

In an earlier chapter, I mentioned a friend of mine who likes to give away books. I also wrote about the first of two books she gave me that dramatically changed my life. The second such book was Watchman Nee's--The Normal Christian Life. In this easy to read, yet profound, book, the Chinese pastor and author explains what should characterize the "normal" Christian life. Striving is replaced by abiding in Christ. Nee's eloquent teaching greatly influenced my studies of Romans six through eight and now shape the content of this chapter.

In our human pride, we desire to make ourselves worthy, and yet such efforts are *chasing after the wind*, as Solomon repeatedly says in Ecclesiastes.[cxxviii] In Romans chapter 7, the great Apostle Paul speaks in a surprising fashion of his tremendous attempts to make himself worthy through self-effort and the repeated frustration and failure such efforts brought. In the end, he passionately declares, *What a wretched man I am!*[cxxix]

Within the modern mindset of self-esteem, valued above all else, awareness of self-wretchedness is to be avoided at all costs. As a result, people tend to react to Paul's declaration of wretchedness by assuming he is just very frustrated by failing yet again. We can all relate to and take comfort from that assumption. If the amazing Apostle Paul struggled with sin to that degree, then maybe I am not so bad after all. I just need to redouble my efforts and keep fighting the good fight.

However, in the study of chapters six through eight, it becomes evident that Paul did not intend to comfort us so that we might continue in our struggle with the flesh, nor was his exclamation of wretchedness an expression of frustration with the intent to renew his efforts. To the

---

[cxxviii] Ecclesiastes 1:16-18; 2:22-26
[cxxix] Romans 7:24 (ESV)

contrary, he is sharing the process of how he came to realize that not a single good thing lives in his flesh.[cxxx] Nada. Nothing!

At the point of Paul's awareness of his complete wretchedness, he finally asks the right question and discovers the blessed truth that he wants all of us to know. He asks, *Who will rescue me from this body that is subject to death*? The answer immediately follows, and I can picture the apostle with hands raised as he triumphantly shouted the answer-- *Thanks be to God, who delivers me through Jesus Christ our Lord!*[cxxxi]

The flesh does not need a twelve-step program. Paul is not saying to try harder but instead to cease all striving and rest in Christ's righteousness. Who we are in ourselves is hopelessly flawed and cannot be fixed. The only answer is to replace the old man with a brand new one that is IN CHRIST.[cxxxii] Then, in Christ, we have everything we need for life and godliness.[cxxxiii] In Christ we are forgiven, cleansed, justified, sanctified, loved, and so on and so on! In Christ, we are dead to sin and alive to righteousness.[cxxxiv] These are the truths of Christ-esteem.

It might seem strange to think that truly realizing your wretchedness is the first step to inner peace. Just think about it though. The world's mantras of how wonderful we are contradict the glaring reality we confront every day. We know that we are deeply flawed. This is why humans struggle endlessly with gaining inner confidence or satisfaction.

When we, instead, recognize our complete inadequacy and as a result look to the Spirit to make true of us what is true of Him, the pressure ends. We are loved and accepted because of Christ, and because God's love is not based on what WE do, it never changes. It is

---

[cxxx] Romans 7:18
[cxxxi] Romans 7:25(ESV)
[cxxxii] 2 Corinthians 5:17 *Therefore, if anyone is in Christ, he is a new creation. The old has passed away; behold, the new has come.* (ESV)
[cxxxiii] 2 Peter 1:3
[cxxxiv] Romans 6:6

not up to us to be worthy. In Christ, we are infinitely worthy. By the blood of Christ, we are worthy whether we have a good day or a bad day, and whether we fail or succeed.

I once lived with a consuming desire for personal perfection, and as a result of all my striving, I had a long list of impressive accomplishments. Yet, the torment of my failures, faults, and limitations, as well as the voices from my past, proved ruthless slave drivers. No matter how hard I tried, I could never be good enough.

Ironically, blessed internal peace came with the awareness that *I know that nothing good dwells in me, that is, in my flesh.*[cxxxv] The truth is (and I knew it well) that in the flesh, Marci is mean, selfish, quick to anger, bossy, weak, prone to depression, and the list goes on and on. But, in Christ, I am righteous and have all that I need to live the Christian life. God's endless words of love, acceptance, and worth ring true and unchanging. When I chose to let go of the constant striving and instead chose to abide in Christ, oh, what peace filled my heart. I too could lift my hands to the heavens and shout, *Thanks be to God, who delivers me through Jesus Christ our Lord!*

Inner Peace Brings Healing

One of my sisters-in-law married into our family later in life. I will never forget sitting at my parents' dining room table, on the occasion of her first holiday dinner with us when Becky shared with me her story of healing. With her blessing, I will now share her story with you.

Raised by her mother and a stepfather who served in the military, my sister-in-law grew up moving from base to base around the world. Her birth father's absence from five years of age forward left a gaping hole in her heart. Although her upbringing made her capable and independent, deep insecurities permeated her being. She chose nursing as a vocation, which allowed one hurting soul to minister to the needs

---

[cxxxv] Romans 7:18(ESV)

of others. As an adult, the Lord called her to salvation in Jesus Christ in February of 1986. Involvement in the church soon became an integral part of her new life in Christ.

In the spring of 2001, Becky developed Rheumatoid Arthritis (RA), the auto-immune disorder that attacks the joints and connective tissues of the body. Appropriate medical treatment began. She did what many Christians do when physical trials arise--counter the pain with personal drive and lots of prayer in an attempt to rise above it. After all, life must go on. As expected, the disease persisted.

In early 2004, a Christian counselor discussed with Becky the possibility that her RA had developed in response to her emotional and spiritual wounds. More specifically, the counselor suggested that as Becky continually berated herself for her inadequacies, her body internally responded by beginning to attack itself. The counselor's theory on her illness brought about a huge "aha" moment. Becky acknowledged the sin of her wrong thinking, and they both prayed for her healing.

A transforming of her mind by the truth began. She began allowing God to replace her self-hatred with His love and full acceptance based on Christ's work on her behalf rather than on her own efforts. No longer was everything dependent on her attempts to be perfect.

Shortly before the counselor's insight, Becky's pastor, noticing her tender heart for others born out of a lifetime of personal hurts and struggles, asked her to consider going through a nine-month training program to become a lay-counselor for their church. She agreed but was concerned about whether or not the Rheumatoid Arthritis would allow her to sit in class for three hours during the week and six hours on Saturdays. She would soon find out that God had the matter in hand.

Choosing to trust God with her concerns over the lengthy sitting required, she began the lay-counseling classes a few weeks later. A few months into the training, while sitting in class, she noticed that a ring had fallen off her finger. Because of the significant swelling and distortion of the joints in her fingers due to RA, that ring had been stuck on her finger for some time. Surprised, she began to inspect her hands and observed a significant change from the typical inflammation. She also realized that she was pain-free and began to move about to evaluate whether or not she truly was without pain. It dawned on her that she had not been aware of pain for some time and could not remember the last time she had taken her meds or refilled her prescription.

With hesitant excitement, she set up an appointment with the doctor and asked for her blood work to be rerun to test for RA factors. After a physical examination and blood results, the doctor said she did not understand it, but Becky appeared to be in full remission. That remission continues to the time of this writing more than fourteen years later.

Please do not think that I am insinuating by Becky's story that autoimmune disease always occurs when spiritual and emotional turmoil causes the physical body to attack itself. I honestly do not know. I can only testify to the link between self-hatred, guilt, and perfectionism in my sister-in-law's case and the healing that repentance from such things brought to her.

However, considering the below bulleted biblical principles covered in past chapters, it seems wise for those with similar diseases to at least consider such a connection:

- Out of the heart (soul and spirit) flows life. (ch.4 & 5)
- The path of life is peace. (ch.6)
- You can be transformed by the renewing of your mind by truth. (ch.7)
- Since the time of Christ, sanctification and healing have gone together. (ch.8)
- Resting in God's love brings joy and health. (ch.9)

The Physical Impact of Guilt

How sad it is that guilt and shame continue to plague the hearts of so many whom Christ has made clean. Frequently in the Psalms King David spoke of the toll guilt takes on the whole body. Take, for example, Psalm 38:4-8 where he said,

My guilt has overwhelmed me like a burden too heavy to bear. My wounds fester and are loathsome because of my sinful folly. I am bowed down and brought very low; all day long I go about mourning. My back is filled with searing pain; there is no health in my body. I am feeble and utterly crushed; I groan in anguish of heart.

Did you notice the clear picture David portrays of his heart stealing life from his entire body because of sin and the resulting heavy burden of guilt? He lists the body's failure to heal, a lack of strength, and horrible back pain as symptoms. Often people read such verses and assume the use of a poetic style means the words are not to be taken literally. What if this assumption is incorrect? Have not the Bible and science both born witness to disease often resulting from a heart without peace?

Consider just one of the three symptoms David mentions that arose from his burden of guilt--back pain. Doctors remain mystified over the reality that the presence of structural problems in the back, such as bulging or herniated discs, stenosis, and disc degeneration, frequently do not match a patient's pain levels. People often have no pain with significant back issues, while others with the same issues have all-consuming pain. Many scientific studies have been completed to shed light on this puzzling fact.

For example, the *New England Journal of Medicine* published a clinical study of the MRI results of ninety-eight people of various ages and sex who were chosen to participate in the study specifically because they reported having absolutely no back pain. Surprisingly, 62% of those individuals showed some form of spine problem and many of them had multiple discs affected.[62] Numerous post-mortem MRI studies also show similar results.

One conclusion from this body of evidence is that *discovering various structural problems in the back may be coincidental to the pain itself.*[cxxxvi] Perhaps such results indicate that non-physical factors (spiritual and emotional) can trigger the onset of pain or determine the degree of pain associated with back problems. Friend, this is huge! If you suffer with significant back pain, please do not ignore these clinical conclusions. Yes, you may have true, structural issues that are known causes of pain, but science shows that something more than physiology influences whether or not you experience that pain and to what degree.

Letting Go of Guilt

Generally, people with pain and illness never consider the possibility that the guilt they carry like a ball and chain might be at the center of their suffering. The world offers little remedy for a heart weighed down by the destructive forces of guilt, but Christianity does. Although unpleasant, guilt has one godly purpose--to bring people to repentance so that cleansing can occur.

Once we have confessed and repented of our sins, we can and should immediately *draw near to God with a sincere heart and with the full assurance that faith brings, having our hearts sprinkled to cleanse us from a guilty conscience and having our bodies washed with pure water* (Hebrews 10:22). Before continuing, take a few moments to read back through each individual phrase of that verse and meditate on those precious words.

As in the ceremony of cleansing when the priest sprinkled the healed leper with the living bird dipped in the shed blood and water, so too our hearts have been sprinkled with the blood of Christ to cleanse

---

[cxxxvi] After citing numerous other clinical studies, as well as their own results, the abstract concluded with, *Given the high prevalence of these findings and of back pain, the discovery by MRI of bulges or protrusions in people with low back pain may frequently be coincidental.*

our guilty consciences. Furthermore, as symbolized by the use of the bird in the ceremony, the Holy Spirit bears witness to the adequacy of the blood for cleansing.

Because of Christ, your Creator declares: "You are clean; you are clean; you are clean; you are clean; you are clean; you are clean; you are clean." Seven times the Judge of the universe repeats, "You are clean!" He does this, not for emphasis, but to demonstrate the totality of cleansing. The Judge is completely satisfied by the blood of Christ.

So many times, after I have sinned and truly repented, Satan tempts me to withdraw from the Lord. "You don't deserve to call yourself a daughter of the King!" the Accuser rails. "You need to punish yourself for a time before your Father will love you again. You will never conquer this sin! You have blown it too many times, and you'll never be any different." Satan speaks what my heart already feels, and so the condemnation could easily take up residence were it not for one thing. Truth. God's Word must dictate my heart's responses, and the truth of that Word is clear.

- *If we confess our sins, he is faithful and just and will forgive us our sins and purify us from all unrighteousness.* (1John 1:9)

- *As far as the east is from the west, so far has he removed our transgressions from us.* (Psalm 103:12)

- *Therefore, there is now NO condemnation for those who are IN CHRIST Jesus.* (Romans 8:1, emphasis mine)

But what if our sin seriously hurts others? What then? I know very well the heart-struggle that results, for such was the case with me. I caused serious harm while unaware of the true nature of muscle testing and allergy treatments (NAET). Upon realizing the demonic nature of those practices and my culpability in hurting some of those I tried to help, my guilt became overwhelming.

How could I possibly accept forgiveness? Surely, I must carry that guilt forever and just hide under a rock, so to speak, because God could never use someone like me. I will never forget one day, though, as I contemplated such thoughts while on my daily walk. The Holy Spirit recalled to my troubled mind the apostle Paul. Before Christ appeared to him on the road to Damascus, this man, who wrote much of the New Testament and who spread the Gospel to the Gentile world, also passionately pursued the imprisonment and death of Christians. If God forgave Paul and greatly used the source of such ghastly sin, then the loving Father will forgive and use me and all others who humbly turn to Him. David spoke a great truth when he said, *Blessed is he whose transgressions are forgiven, whose sins are covered. Blessed is the man whose sin the LORD does not count against him.*[cxxxvii] Do I hear an "Amen!"?

Believing Truth When Hearts Condemn

1 John 3:19-21 comes to mind when I think about how to handle the hearts continued condemnation following repentance. *This is how we know that we belong to the truth and how we set our hearts at rest in his presence: If our hearts condemn us, we know that God is greater than our hearts, and he knows everything.* God is greater than our hearts! To restore peace within, we must choose to believe God's truth over our feelings. God is not ignorant of the gravity of a particular sin. He knows everything, and He says that the blood of Christ is sufficient for ALL sin. Paul has a powerful reminder for us when Satan or any person attempts to convince us otherwise.

> *Who will bring any charge against those whom God has chosen? It is God who justifies. Who then is the one who condemns? No one. Christ Jesus who died—more than that, who was raised to*

[cxxxvii] Psalm 32:1-2

life—is at the right hand of God and is also interceding for us. [cxxxviii]

When Satan tempts you to believe the voices from the past, consciously choose to counter them with, "but God says..." I have placed some Scriptures in Appendix D that speak of who you are in Christ and how God views you. Perhaps they can be a resource to help you take captive wrong thinking and form new, healthy patterns of thought. Meditate on those truths.

A New Creation

In summary, Christ-esteem impacts two primary ways in which you view yourself: First, God's Word alone holds the truth about your worth, value, and significance IN Christ. Second, in Christ, you are a new creation, free of guilt because Jesus' blood satisfies God. Because the Lord Almighty loves and values you, He alone makes you worthy through His Son, Jesus Christ. **Peace with yourself comes from believing God's truth about you and brings health to your whole body**. You are the righteousness of God! Go in peace, my friend.

———————————

Biblical Principle: *Peace with myself comes from believing God's truth about me and brings health to my whole body.*

Call to Action: *Take some time to worship the Lord with a thankful heart for all that He has accomplished for you.*

———————————

[cxxxviii] Romans 8:33-34

CHAPTER 16

Peace With Others

Follow God's example, therefore, as dearly loved children and walk in the way of love, just as Christ loved us and gave himself up for us as a fragrant offering and sacrifice to God.
Ephesians 5:1-2

Testifying to the joy of spring, the birds joined the chorus of Elvine Johannessen as she twirled about the kitchen in her flowing, pink dress with a sash. Oh, how she had longed for just one pretty dress to wear. As the Norwegian wife of a humble minister during the early 1900s and living on the lonely farmlands of Wisconsin, practical black or gray dresses typically adorned her feminine frame.

At twenty-three, she had only an infant and cows to talk to while her husband endlessly studied theology, preached, and ministered to the needs of his poor, immigrant congregation. She was content but for one thing--Elvine dreamt of feeling pretty in a flowing dress with a sash. After first scrimping pennies so her husband might have a greatly needed lamp for study at night, she had finally saved enough to justify making her private dream a reality. The occasion warranted unpinning her tightly bound hair to let it swirl about her face just as the dress did about her legs. Her husband came into the room, and she twirled to face him, wrongfully anticipating a pleased reaction.

Moments later the delicate pink fabric, now torn to pieces, littered the kitchen floor, and the pounding of horse hooves down the lane as her husband left the yard punctuated the anger rising up in Elvine's heart. How could he be so cruel as to destroy her one frivolity? She wept long and loud as she gathered the remnants of her dream and placed them in a box, determined to keep them as a memorial of the injustice committed. She resolutely decided she would never forgive the man she once loved. She then fixed her mind on contriving a plan to leave him.

This true story, as originally told by Elvine's daughter, Margaret Jensen, in *First We Have Coffee*, continues on to describe her mother's intention to approach a traveling preacher with the evidence of her husband's sin against her. Surely, once the pastor heard the story, he would help the young wife to take a train back to her family in New York.

Oblivious to the pain he had caused by his outburst, her husband went on with life as always. For Elvine, though, the internal joy, once so characteristic, was pushed aside to make room for the bitterness that now crowded her soul. With the visiting minister's imminent arrival, she thought through every detail of how she might approach him for a private audience. The occasion must follow the Sunday service.

Sitting on the hard pew of their rural church on the Sunday of the visiting preacher's visit, Elvine had no desire to surrender her obsessive thoughts in order to listen. Nonetheless, the pastor's reading of Mark 11:25 broke through. *And when you stand praying, if you hold anything against anyone, forgive them, so that your Father in heaven may forgive you your sins.* Panic welled up in her as God's Word pierced a hole in her bitter resolve. "Some things just cannot be forgiven!" she thought, but the minister seemed to read her mind as his sermon continued.

When you forgive, you must destroy the evidence, and remember only to love. "For God so loved the world that he gave his only begotten Son, that whosoever believeth in Him should not perish, but have everlasting life." *In closing, let us stand and say the Lord's prayer.* *"Forgive us our debts, as we forgive our debtors."*[63]

The Spirit's quiet prodding of Elvine's heart brought many tears on the trip home. She knew what she must do, but as she pulled the shredded dress from the box, a battle raged in her heart. *True forgiveness destroys the evidence*, echoed so loudly in her conscience that she failed to hear her husband's approach from behind while the dress caught fire in the wood-burning stove.

"What are you doing?" he asked.
Trembling with sobs, she said, "I am destroying the evidence."
To herself, she said, "My offering to God."
Then he remembered! Pale and shaken, he murmured, "Please forgive me."[64]

Because this young woman chose to heed the Holy Spirit's conviction and forgive, she and her husband went on to decades of fruitful ministry and to raise numerous children who also grew up to serve the Lord themselves. Oh, what a tremendous loss she and countless others would have suffered if she had chosen to harbor bitterness rather than forgive.

Forgiveness

Who has not been significantly hurt by others? Not to make light of a profound problem, but a universal reality of living in a sin-cursed world is that mortals wound mortals. As discussed in the chapters on the heart, **out of the heart (soul and spirit) flows life.** Therefore, when emotional injuries inflicted by others are allowed to fester, rather than heal, the physical impact can be significant. Forgiveness is the oh, so difficult act necessary to prevent anger, hatred, and bitterness from taking up residence in the heart--our source for life.

As you stand praying, forgive. To one who has been wronged, those five straightforward words will likely unleash a torrent of emotion and struggle at their impossibility. How does one forgive the unforgivable? Truthfully, it is indeed an impossible task, and yet one the Lord requires of us.

A Lesson From Job

The book of Job came up in the previous chapter, and I wish to make a further observation about it here. His unshakable trust in God in the midst of an onslaught of unbearable tragedies has stood as a powerful testimony throughout the ages. Countless times I have read the book of Job and gained insight and encouragement while undergoing times of suffering, but only this last time of reading it did I notice a remarkable detail at the end of the story.

Thirty-six of the forty-two chapters in the book of Job contain a conversation between Job and his so-called friends. Back and forth the men went, giving long-winded speeches that insisted on Job being at fault for the catastrophes that befell him, and the suffering God allowed to be brought upon him. In spite of Job's unimaginable anguish, the well-intentioned men ceaselessly asserted that he should repent from his wrongdoing. I cannot fathom the depths of anger and resentment Job surely felt as their words poured forth like acid on an open wound.

Sarcasm dripped from Job's words in response to their long-winded speeches revealing the injury they caused. *Doubtless, you are the only people who matter, and wisdom will die with you. But I have a mind as well as you; I am not inferior to you.*[cxxxix] And, yet the condemning speeches continued, and Job's pain intensified. His anger at the injustice of their words rings loud and clear in the following passage:

[cxxxix] Job 12:2-3

How long will you torment me and crush me with words? Ten times now you have reproached me; shamelessly you attack me. If it is true that I have gone astray, my error remains my concern alone. If indeed you would exalt yourselves above me and use my humiliation against me, then know that God has wronged me and drawn his net around me.[cxl]

Finally, God interrupted their injurious speeches and spoke directly to Job. Following the Almighty's discourse, God harshly rebuked the other men present for their ignorant words against His faithful servant. Then comes a noteworthy aspect of this story that I only recently came to consider significant. See if you pick up on it from these verses:

So now take seven bulls and seven rams and go to my servant Job and sacrifice a burnt offering for yourselves. My servant Job will pray for you, and I will accept his prayer and not deal with you according to your folly. You have not spoken the truth about me, as my servant Job has."... and the Lord accepted Job's prayer. After Job had prayed for his friends, the Lord restored his fortunes and gave him twice as much as he had before.[cxli]

Before God would heal Job and restore all of his wealth, blessing him with double of that which he had previously, God required Job to pray for the very men who had just wronged him. Why? Based on other Scriptures that warn against bitterness, it would appear that the Lord did not want His righteous servant to become bitter towards those who had wounded him.[cxlii] Forgiveness was needed. It is only after Job's prayers for his undeserving friends that the Bible describes a time of restored health, and fellowship between him, his family, and friends. Bitterness, anger, and unforgiveness ruin relationships, and the Lord desires that His children live in peace and fellowship with others.

[cxl] Job 19:2-6
[cxli] Job 42:8-10
[cxlii] Deuteronomy 29:18 & Hebrews 12:15

The Glory of God

According to my journal, a year ago (August of 2017) I pleaded with the Lord that He might reveal Himself afresh to me --"to show me His glory." A sermon I had heard a few days earlier prompted the request. The pastor had spoken from Exodus 33, which tells of a private conversation between Moses and the LORD sometime after the first giving of the ten commandments. Following the disastrous incident with the golden calf, Moses must have felt an inundation of conflicting emotions--anger at the people's rebelliousness, sorrow at the harsh discipline their actions required, and a tremendous inadequacy for the task of leading such an obstinate bunch.

So, before going up the mountain once again in order to receive the law of God, Moses said to the LORD, *If you are pleased with me, teach me your ways so I may know you and continue to find favor with you. Remember that this nation is your people...Now show me your glory.* [cxliii]

What aspect of God's character do you suppose constitutes His glory? Is it His power or perhaps His holiness? Let us look at God's response to Moses for our answer.

> *And he passed in front of Moses, proclaiming, "The Lord, the Lord, the compassionate and gracious God, slow to anger, abounding in love and faithfulness, maintaining love to thousands, and forgiving wickedness, rebellion, and sin.* [cxliv]

In Psalm 103, David references this story of Moses' request to see God's glory but then elaborates further.[cxlv] The Psalm speaks in great detail of how the loving Father remembers our human frailties and treats us accordingly, casts our sins as far as the east is from the west,

---

[cxliii] Exodus 33:13 & 18
[cxliv] Exodus 34:6-7
[cxlv] Compare Exodus 34:6 to Psalm 103:8.

and shows His love from one generation to the next. Rather than some majestic display of power or beauty, the glory of God is the undeserved depth of love and compassion that God exhibits toward His people. The truth of God's glory undergirds every aspect of His work throughout time.

When Moses asked to see God's glory, the Almighty said that He must cover Moses' view as the glory of God passed by because no one could see the face of God.[cxlvi] However, with the arrival of Jesus Christ, the mystery of God's glory was finally revealed for all mankind to see. *The Word became flesh and made his dwelling among us. We have seen his glory, the glory of the one and only Son, who came from the Father, full of grace and truth.[cxlvii]* Jesus said that anyone who saw Him had seen the Father.[cxlviii]

Now think about this: If God's glory is His compassion, love, graciousness, forgiveness, and not treating people according to what their sins deserve, then, of course, Christ is the face of that glory! What the Father hid from Moses and the prophets of old, He revealed in the flesh when Jesus came to the earth as a man to die in the place of sinners.

Paul spoke much of knowing the mystery of Christ. What is this mystery? Colossians 1:25-27 provides the answer.

> *I have become its servant by the commission God gave me to present to you the word of God in its fullness—the mystery that has been kept hidden for ages and generations but is now disclosed to the Lord's people. To them, God has chosen to make known among the Gentiles the glorious riches of this mystery, which is Christ in you, the hope of glory.*

Not only has the Father revealed His love (glory) through Christ, but His mysterious plan from the beginning was to reveal His glory as

---

[cxlvi] Exodus 33:20
[cxlvii] John 1:14
[cxlviii] John 14:9

Christ shines forth THROUGH US! So, how do we glorify the Father? Surely, the hope of glory is seen every time we show compassion and graciousness to the undeserving. When we forgive as Christ forgave us, we radiate His glory. So too, when we choose to overlook an offense, God is glorified.[cxlix]

Therefore, as God's chosen people, holy and dearly loved, clothe yourselves with compassion, kindness, humility, gentleness and patience. Bear with each other and forgive one another if any of you has a grievance against someone. Forgive as the Lord forgave you. And over all these virtues put on love, which binds them all together in perfect unity. Let the peace of Christ rule in your hearts, since as members of one body you were called to peace. And be thankful. Let the message of Christ dwell among you richly...

Oh, but this is where I so often stumble and fall. I do not want to overlook an offense or love those who reject me or forgive wrongs that wound me deeply or... In fact, I cannot do it, and neither can you! Only when we allow the love of Christ dwelling in us to shape our thoughts, desires, and actions can we glorify the Father in our day-to-day life. Therein lies our next biblical principle of health: **God's love filling your heart must motivate you towards peace with others, bringing health and healing to your whole person.** What is your heart? Is it to glorify the Father? Then let the love the Father has lavished on you flow over into the lives of others, especially the undeserving. Upon doing so, your heart at peace will give life to your body.

After pleading a year ago with God to show me His glory, He answered by opening my eyes to the nature of His glory. However, in God's typical practice of revealing truth and then requiring application, He almost immediately unearthed my repeated attempts at burying a decade of heartache so that I might forgive a particular individual who

---

[cxlix] Proverbs 19:11

had repeatedly rejected me. The Father insisted that it would be in the very act of loving this one who did not deserve my forgiveness and certainly not my love that I would see God's glory. I needed to destroy the evidence (cast their sin as far as the east is from the west). Then, while I stood praying, forgive, and remember only to love. How could I possibly do such a thing? No longer I but Christ! This is the mystery of God.

Cats or People?

Love your neighbor as yourself.[cl]   In only five words Jesus summarized the teaching of much of the New Testament. The verse that precedes that simple command speaks of loving the Lord with every part of our being. It is then, out of the Father's love that we can love both ourselves and others. It is quite simple, really, and yet so very difficult.

After God opened my eyes to His unfailing and unconditional love for me in 2008, I found myself wanting to stay in a safe circle that included only me, the Lord, and my family. Nestled in the cleft of my Savior's love, I found what my soul had been searching for--security, love, acceptance, hope, significance, and the list goes on and on.

However, involvement with others opened up the possibility of further rejection, hurt, criticism, cruelty, and the list goes on and on. Not to mention, it is just so much easier to be holy when one does not have to deal with the annoyances of others. The choice seemed quite simple, and for a time, God allowed me to draw near only to Him as He tended to and bound up my broken heart.

During that time my cats were my faithful companions. Every morning Patches, a large, white cat with a couple of big, black spots would drape himself around my head while I sat in a recliner to have my devotions. Like a dog, he followed me around the house as though his sole desire was to be with me. Another cat, C.C., named such

---

[cl] Luke 10:27

because he was my son, Caleb's cat, had always had an uncanny sense of when his owners were troubled or sick. His long hair and quiet presence brought us much comfort for eighteen years. I found myself frequently thinking about how much better cats were than people. Life was safe and good as long as I kept people at bay.

But then God took away my kitties. Both died within a short time of each other. Greatly saddened by the loss, I set about to acquire new feline companions but to no avail. In a year's time, we lost five cats. It became clear that God desired for me to be involved in the lives of His people and would continue to prevent me from the blessing of cats as long as I persisted in seeking the safety of seclusion. The time had come for me to *follow God's example, therefore, as dearly loved children and walk in the way of love, just as Christ loved us and gave himself up for us as a fragrant offering and sacrifice to God.*[cli]

The Father did not send His only begotten Son to die for animals or things but for people. People, as imperfect and lowly as they are, occupy the center of God's focus and plan throughout time. The apostle John goes into great detail about how our love for others is THE defining trait of the true believer. *This is how we know we are in him. Whoever claims to live in him must live as Jesus did. Anyone who claims to be in the light but hates a brother or sister is still in the darkness.*[clii]

The Glory of God in the Church

With internet access, anyone can listen to the most gifted preachers and teachers of God's Word from the safety and comfort of a location of their choosing. No longer must Christians suffer through worship services containing anything, not to their liking, such as a preacher who has not yet discovered how to entertain the masses while teaching sound doctrine. Never again must one endure Betty and Fred,

---

[cli] Ephesians 5:1-2
[clii] 1 John 2:5-6 & 9

who can be so annoying or Jim and Martha, who never stop complaining or Tom and Jane, who judge everyone but themselves or... Instead, Christians can worship and learn about God without so many difficult people distracting them. Besides, they are all just hypocrites anyway, right?

But here is the problem with such thinking. Hebrews 10:25-27 says, quite explicitly, that we are to actually gather regularly with believers:

> *not giving up meeting together, as some are in the habit of doing, but encouraging one another—and all the more as you see the Day approaching. If we deliberately keep on sinning after we have received the knowledge of the truth, no sacrifice for sins is left, but only a fearful expectation of judgment and of raging fire that will consume the enemies of God.*

The model God set forth from Acts to Revelation clearly communicates an expectation that each individual who has placed their faith in Christ personally participate with a local body of believers. The picture laid out in Acts 2 describes close fellowship among Christians as they learn from God's Word, eat together, encourage one another, pray for each other, and share in communion as the bride of Christ. Furthermore, 1 Corinthians 12 details how each individual in the body of Christ has been spiritually gifted to minister specifically within that body. It leaves no ambiguity regarding the importance of functioning as a unified body where each does his part.[cliii]

So, despite the convenience of online, television, or radio services, God's plan mandates worship in the context of fellowship. I know that it can be exceedingly difficult to find a church that fits well with individual preferences and that remains doctrinally sound. I also know the tremendous pain that believers within the church sometimes cause. However, to neglect the local church and God's design for His children to function within that body is to walk in sin. It really is that simple,

---

[cliii] 1 Corinthians 12:7-27

and every believer must purpose never to cease from seeking the fellowship of other believers.

The exquisite plan of God from the beginning of time included that He would glorify Himself through His Son dwelling in individuals, who then corporately demonstrate the love, compassion, and grace of God to an undeserving world. In these harsh times, where criticism of Christians abounds, the church provides a blessed haven of love and support. Dear brother or sister in Christ, do not abandon the beauty of God's perfect plan to glorify himself through His people working together in love and unity.

Healing Promised

Biblical fasting is a practice I recommend for times of humbly and earnestly seeking God, and Isaiah 58 describes how God desires that fasting, as well as daily life, should reflect the Father's love for people. Do you want God to hear your prayers for healing? Then, love others the passage says. I know it is long, but you must read it for yourself.

> *Is not this the kind of fasting I have chosen: to loose the chains of injustice and untie the cords of the yoke, to set the oppressed free and break every yoke?*

> *Is it not to share your food with the hungry and to provide the poor wanderer with shelter—when you see the naked, to clothe them, and not to turn away from your own flesh and blood?*

> *Then your light will break forth like the dawn, and your healing will quickly appear; then your righteousness will go before you, and the glory of the Lord will be your rear guard. Then you will call, and the Lord will answer; you will cry for help, and he will say: Here am I.*

> *"If you do away with the yoke of oppression, with the pointing finger and malicious talk, and if you spend yourselves in behalf of the hungry and satisfy the needs of the oppressed, then your*

light will rise in the darkness, and your night will become like the noonday.

The Lord will guide you always; he will satisfy your needs in a sun-scorched land and will strengthen your frame. You will be like a well-watered garden, like a spring whose waters never fail.[cliv]

Similar passages also link the Lord's healing to our outward expressions of love and compassion for others with the Lord bringing healing. Perhaps you recall my explanation of the word "refresh" from Peter's sermon following the healing of the lame man. In Proverbs 11:17 & 25, we see an Old Testament use of the word. *Those who are kind benefit themselves, but the cruel bring ruin on themselves. A generous person will prosper; whoever refreshes others will be refreshed.*

Another place where God links a promise of healing to showing compassion for others comes from Psalm 41:3-4.

Blessed are those who have regard for the weak; the Lord delivers them in times of trouble. The Lord protects and preserves them—they are counted among the blessed in the land—he does not give them over to the desire of their foes. The Lord sustains them on their sickbed and restores them from their bed of illness. I said, "Have mercy on me, Lord heal me, for I have sinned against you."

If we desire to live according to the will of the Lord, then we must model His heart and His actions by loving others at home, in the church, and in the world. Peace with others is so much more than ridding oneself of a heart of bitterness, although that clearly tops the list.[clv] Peace with others encompasses who we are intended to be in

---

[cliv] Isaiah 58:6-11

[clv] Hebrews 12:14-15 *Make every effort to live in peace with everyone and to be holy; without holiness no one will see the Lord. See to it that no one falls*

Christ and the very plan of God to glorify Himself. *We know that we have passed from death to life because we love each other. Anyone who does not love remains in death.*[clvi]

Have you been walking in darkness? It is time to come into the light. If you lack peace in your heart towards others, you also undoubtedly suffer from health issues or will before long. As you stand praying, forgive. Ask the Lord to totally replace any hurt, anger, and bitter poison crowding your soul with the love the Father has lavished on you. Then you too will see the glory of God.

Biblical Principle: *God's love filling your heart must motivate you towards peace with others, bringing health and healing to your whole person.*

Call to Action: *Make a list of the people in your past and present whose remembrance calls hurt and anger to mind. Begin praying that God will change your heart that you might forgive as Christ forgave you and that you may remember only to love. If you have not been an active part of a local body of believers, repent and prayerfully seek to walk in obedience.*

---

short of the grace of God and that no bitter root grows up to cause trouble and defile many.
[clvi] 1 John 3:14-15

CHAPTER 17

Spiritual Forces & Health

For we do not wrestle against flesh and blood, but against the rulers, against the authorities, against the cosmic powers over this present darkness, against the spiritual forces of evil in the heavenly places. Ephesians 6:12 ESV

"Marci, you need to see this email right away," my husband said with concern as I entered the front door of my house.

Emails from my website came with some regularity, but apparently, this one was more concerning than most.

It read, "May I please call you? I so much need to speak with you about a heart-breaking situation that just occurred. We found your website about two weeks ago, and all hell has broken loose since then."

Pausing to pray for wisdom that I might rightly respond to whatever story this stranger had to tell, I then picked up the phone. An hour and many shared tears later, I closed the call with prayer and, with a heavy heart, said goodbye. The dear sister in the Lord with whom I spoke had shared the tragic story of her family's involvement with a young man that her eldest son had befriended. They had generously shared the love of Christ in word and in deed with him over the course of a year. He was full of promise, although he had yet to decide to trust Jesus as his Savior.

One evening after eating dinner at their house, the young man described to them a pain in his chest that seemed to come on him whenever he tried to read the Bible. He told them how his mother was proficient in Body Code, one of the many alternative health practices that utilize muscle testing and that she used it frequently in his home. So, when this pain would arise, he would ask her to "treat" him, following which the pain would immediately subside. As he described this to the Christian mother of his friend, she felt with certainty the Holy Spirit's prompting that this was demonic and told him so. To the surprise of all, he readily agreed, and said he was done with it all. She warned him not to ever have the "treatment" done again.

A short time later the pain again came on him with great intensity, and so he asked his mother to treat him once again. Apparently, it is one thing to be an ignorant participant, but quite another to know of Satan's work and seek it for help. His personality changed suddenly and dramatically. He began describing to others that he felt tormented, and thoughts of suicide consumed him. He began texting disturbing pictures related to his plans for killing himself.

The Christian family fasted, prayed, and pleaded with him to turn to the Lord for salvation. When he went to this family's home, the daughters, who had written and recorded songs that beautifully spoke of the Gospel, would sing to comfort him. Like with King Saul when David played the harp, this young man's torment would cease with the music. Everything indicated that he had become demon possessed as a result of the "treatment" he had received.

A couple of weeks later, however, he texted his sorrowful, last words to multiple members of their family and then shot and killed himself on a farm tractor.

Satan's Power to Deceive

In an attempt to follow the biblical instruction, *Have nothing to do with the fruitless deeds of darkness, but rather expose them,*[clvii] I wrote a series of three blog articles about my experiences with energy medicine and the conclusions I drew from them. I never anticipated the impact those writings would have.[clviii] Since their posting, I have received a steady flow of emails and phone calls from people, mostly Christian, who have become ensnared by energy medicine. Through their stories, my own experiences, and continued research, I have become aware of the pervasive work of Satan to ensnare Christians who are sick.

The apostle Paul warned that Satan would take this tactic in the end times when he wrote, *The Spirit clearly says that in later times some will abandon the faith and follow deceiving spirits and things taught by demons.*[clix] Jesus also warned that Satan's signs and wonders might also deceive the elect.[clx] The next biblical principle of health comes from those warnings: **Satan uses deception to ensnare Christians through demonically based health practices.** I never dreamed that I would be one of the deceived, but I was.

Relentless, unending pain has a way of making people desperate, and I was no different. Traditional medicine typically fails to provide solutions to chronic conditions, and so people often turn to alternative practices that report bringing relief to many. Unfortunately, it is in this realm that Satan has gained a tremendous foothold in the lives of countless Christians who truly love God.

Because of this ever-increasing problem, I will share what transpired to bring about my conclusions along with eleven red flags (warning signs) to be on the lookout for when considering alternative health practices. Although my involvement was with one application that utilized muscle testing (Applied Kinesiology or AK), I have come

[clvii] Ephesians 5:11
[clviii] For an explanation of muscle testing, as well as links to my articles and audio lesson on AK, see Appendix E.
[clix] 1 Timothy 4:1
[clx] Matthew 24:24-25

to learn of seemingly endless variations on the same practices. Therefore, please do not get bogged down in the specifics, thinking that what you are considering does "this" and not "that," so it must be okay.

Whether an alternative health methodology produces results should never be the deciding factor in whether a Christian should become involved with it. The key issue, rather, revolves around understanding how it works. **Either it produces results by purely physical means, or the results stem from spiritual forces.** Trying to determine this troubled me greatly when I first became involved in alternative medicine. However, an experience involving the apparent healing of my thyroid trumped all other logic, and the gentle voice of the Holy Spirit faded as I dove headlong into the deep waters of energy medicine.

The particular branch of alternative medicine in which I became involved operated under the premise that most chronic health problems are caused by allergies. It taught simple methods for diagnosing those allergies and reprogramming the body to eradicate them. In my experience, the first results of this methodology were dramatic, but those initial experiences gave way to a constant need to retreat previously "cleared" allergies and to treat for the first time every conceivable thing I encountered in life to hold on to my tenuous level of health.

I learned to do it all myself and taught my family members as well so that I could manage my symptoms at home. When treating at home, I sometimes "Christianized" it by praying in place of a questionable part of the process where speaking to the body was done. Surely if there was any cause for concern, praying made it alright, I thought.

By this point, God had healed me of all my traditionally diagnosed conditions, and yet I began constantly reacting in new ways to everything. However, I found that a quick treatment could have me right-as-rain in a couple of minutes. When I say that I reacted to everything, I mean everything from pollen to electricity, and the reactions were often severe and quite bizarre. I would get so weak that I might collapse from stepping on a pile of pollen while walking. The same thing would happen if I walked under streetlights. The time spent testing and treating all these things seemed a small price to pay for the great relief it brought.

As I became quite proficient in muscle testing or AK, I began treating others in what I thought was a ministry to the hurting. During that time, I saw two more instances of apparent miraculous results. One was with a friend's four-month-old baby who had screamed endlessly since she was born and slept very little. By using surrogate testing,[clxi] I determined that the child was allergic to the formula they were feeding her. I then treated the baby through her mother, and she finally stopped screaming and fell asleep.

When I came back the next day, I saw a remarkably changed child. The mother reported that, after I left, her baby had had an enormous bowel movement and then slept for three straight hours for the first time since she was born. I then tested and treated the infant for the second formula they had been using and left. It was reported to me that the same thing happened as before, but this time the baby slept through the entire night for the first time. From the next morning forward, the parents reported that she was a different child, with a sweet disposition.

The other seemingly miraculous case was with a man who had muscular dystrophy as a child, but it had gone into remission as a teenager. Unfortunately, his symptoms were returning, and he was terrified of the outcome. Following my treatment for a granola bar he had started eating every day, the symptoms disappeared. These significant results fueled my certainty of the amazing power of muscle testing and motivated me to disregard several concerns.

Those concerns included the suicide of a close friend following her involvement with AK to treat for bipolar disorder. After treatments

---

[clxi] Surrogate testing is used for those who cannot perform the muscle test-- small children, the elderly, or those who are too weak. The tester pushes down on the surrogate's arm while he or she makes skin contact with the one being tested.

seemed to improve her mental state, she decided to quit taking her medication, following which she spiraled out of control.

A relative by marriage who has ulcerative colitis allowed me to test and treat her, following which she seemed to be no longer allergic to dairy. As is so typical of these treatments, the initial appearance of improvement reversed, but being unaware of this, she continued eating dairy. As a result, she ended up in the hospital for days in grave condition.

I also saw a friend with health issues progress into all-consuming environmental disease following my getting her involved in muscle testing. Within a period of weeks, she became unable to breathe without panic outside of her now heavily controlled home environment, unable to wear anything that had not been meticulously washed under strict controls or eat more than the most basic foods that had been carefully prepared. Her life became a constant torment.

A year and a half into my involvement with AK, a friend spoke to me of my "bondage" to these practices, and I began earnestly seeking the Lord through His Word. Following the weeks I described in an earlier chapter, during which I repented of any sin God brought to my attention, I simply prayed in the quiet of my bedroom and asked God for healing from all my allergic reactions. At that moment, God miraculously healed me, separate from any allergy treatments. I no longer muscle-tested positive for a single allergy. What I now realize is that God merely required the unclean spirits who had been tormenting me to stop.

An Unwanted Presence

Following that day, I never again needed AK personally, but I continued to treat others while earnestly praying that God would continue to reveal any other areas of sin in my life. Some concerning and unexplainable things began happening. I believe that, because of my prayers, significant spiritual warfare began. Just as in the Bible, when Jesus entered the presence of demons, and they became agitated--

doing things that made their presence known, so also the demons once quiet influence became noticeable around me. At least twice, as I specifically remember, doors in my house slammed unexplainably while I was home alone. My son, who also had a tremendous ability for muscle testing, started having frightening "prophetic" dreams.

One particularly bizarre and unexplainable instance unsettled our whole family. We were on vacation in New York, and I wanted to mail out postcards from a local post office to all my nieces and nephews. After addressing the cards while sitting in the idling car, I exited and went inside. When I came back out of the building and again sat in the car, my son began telling me the conversation he and my husband had while I was gone.

I immediately interrupted and finished telling him in great detail about their conversation. Confused, I asked them why they were bothering to repeat a conversation that they knew I had already heard in its entirety. They were both perplexed and insisted repeatedly that there was no way that I could have known the details of their conversation.

They both distinctly remembered watching me wait in line through the glass windows of the post office as they had that conversation. I kept insisting that they were wrong and that they most definitely had the conversation in the car while I addressed the postcards. With mutual expressions of concern and confusion, they reiterated that they had waited in silence for me to exit the car before they began their conversation. How did I hear and know the words spoken in my absence?

Following that incident, I began praying that God would make it clear if I had opened myself and my family up to Satanic influences. I was not ready to admit it to anyone, but I was beginning to suspect that I did not just have an uncanny sensitivity for muscle testing but that I had developed an actual power that could not possibly be explained scientifically. I began noticing that I seemed to know without muscle testing, whether someone would test "allergic" to something. I suspected that this foreknowledge matched up to muscle testing with

100% accuracy but was afraid to test the theory. The ramifications were too frightening.

For the first time, I understood how it is that many practitioners can "muscle test" people on the phone. These clairvoyant abilities defied scientific explanation and pointed to the true source of power. I am ashamed to admit, however, that I liked this sense of power and resisted the thought of giving it up. Eventually, however, I confessed my suspicion of "special knowledge" to my husband and told him that I feared the practices I was involved in were based on spiritual power.

I will never forget the night of that confession. My husband, Seth, devised a way to test the theory of "special knowledge." First, he named things in the room and simply asked me if he was allergic to them. As soon as the object was named an immediate and strong sense of the answer came to me. Perhaps one could compare it with reading a question on a test and immediately knowing, without a doubt, that you know the correct answer. The sense was so strong that it made me want to laugh at the absurdity of it. Before we did any muscle testing, my husband recorded my predictions as to how he would test for well over ten things.

When he finished recording my clairvoyant answers, I muscle tested him and found that 100% of the time, my foreknown answers matched the muscle testing results. (Keep in mind that Seth is a very strong man. When I muscle tested him and he was "allergic," though he tried to resist, I barely had to exert any effort to press his arm down.) After testing in a variety of ways with 100% accuracy, Seth calculated the statistical odds of such occurring by chance. It was staggering!

Afterward, we both just sat, rather stunned. The odds were impossible for me to have correctly guessed every time. Our Christian faith has a term for such predictive power: divination. And divination, the Bible teaches, is never the result of good forces but always of evil.

Now please understand; we are not charismatic in our theological persuasion, and even if I can be swayed by emotions, Seth is a logic, fact-based kind of man. Although as Christians we believe in spiritual forces, we are not of a mentality that sees angels and demons behind every act. Furthermore, we knew that a true believer has the Holy Spirit indwelling them and therefore cannot be possessed by demonic powers.[clxii] It appeared, though, that demonic forces were somehow influencing me outwardly.

We called our son in and explained to him what we believed to be the case. As the spiritual head of our home, Seth prayed for God's protection, and then in the name of Jesus, verbally instructed any demonic forces present that they must get out of our home. When he did so, an indescribable and overwhelming presence of fear and evil encompassed me so pervasively that I could hardly breathe, and I began crying out. Seth again renounced any influence that Satan had on me, and as he did so my fear and physical distress ended.

Peace enveloped us all as we immediately began ridding our house of every bit of literature and paraphernalia related to those practices. However, soon thereafter, I experienced a compelling temptation to rescue the stuff from the trashcan by the street. It was like voices were calling from outside. Recognizing the temptation, I asked Seth to completely eliminate the possibility of retrieving the material, once and for all.

I was afraid to try muscle testing again, but the next day I had to know if perhaps our conclusions about Satan's involvement had been wrong. If my ability was the result of science or even God's, not Satan's power, then I should still be able to muscle test as before. So, I tried one final time, and had absolutely no ability, nor did I have any sort of sense of "special knowledge."

Eleven Red Flags

Most Christians are aware of the strong biblical warnings against divination and witchcraft and abhor the thought of ever being party to such wickedness. [clxiii] Yet, the Deceiver is cunning. Through the ages, he has continually morphed the appearance of divination and witchcraft

---

[clxii] 1 Corinthians 6:19, Romans 8:9-11, 1 John 4:4
[clxiii] Deut. 18:10&14, 2 Chron.33:6, Lev. 19:26, & many others

to ensnare the unsuspecting. Knowing what to look for proves critical
for discerning his latest methods. The critical question to answer is the
following: If the alternative practice works (produces results), does it
do so by physical means or is it only spiritually explainable?

To help determine that answer, I will list eleven things to be on the
lookout for when considering a particular type of alternative or
energetic medicine. For a quick reference guide to a concise list of the
11 red flags, see Appendix F.

**1. Is the information acquired by the practice the result of secret
knowledge?**

Meriam Websters Dictionary defines divination as *the art or
practice that seeks to foresee or foretell future events or discover
hidden knowledge usually by the interpretation of omens or by the aid
of supernatural powers.* Alternative practices that rely on demonic
power to produce results claim that the body can reveal knowledge
about itself that typical scientific tests fail to show. This idea of
gaining hidden knowledge from the body comes from the religious
underpinnings of these practices--that God is in all things. Therefore,
your body is its own separate entity that, as a god, can communicate
mysteriously. These pantheistic ideas are rampant in eastern and new
age religions and the health practices that developed from them.

I have heard from many Christians that they use muscle testing to
make their every decision. The availability of this method as a
replacement for the Holy Spirit's guidance clearly reveals it as
divination. If the Holy Spirit worked in such ways, God would have
instructed us about this in His Word.

**2. Do you have a sense of unease (lack peace) when you think
about the practice?**

Many people who contact me about these practices indicate that,
although they did not know why, they had a sense that something did

not seem right about the alternative practice they were considering or using. As Christians, we have the indwelling Holy Spirit to guide us into truth and to convict us of sin. His presence brings life and peace. If these are missing, then it is good to ask why.

3. Have the results of alternative testing been verified through traditionally accepted methods (blood tests, x-rays, etc.) or do the alternative methods contradict traditional results?

Practitioners who use muscle testing or other divination techniques to diagnose conditions are quick to dismiss traditional results in favor of their own because they believe "the body doesn't lie." They guide their patients into unverified, expensive, and all-consuming protocols based on unproven testing that only leads to downward spiraling health. However, because patients have enough "good days" to encourage them, they stay the course and never truly get better.

If indeed a purely physical explanation for AK and its various branches exists, then double-blind studies should demonstrate consistent, reproducible results. Numerous studies have shown that this is not the case.[65] One such study, done in 2014 tested fifty-one people by three respected AK practitioners-one male and two female. They also tested the subjects using a hand dynamometer with no practitioner present.[clxiv] AK claims that the body recognizes things by their "energy" and reveals that knowledge through muscle strength. This subtle energy is perceived through touch, and so the subjects were tested by all three practitioners and the dynamometer while holding two vials, one at a time--one containing a clear liquid containing a lethal concentration of a toxin and the other containing a saline solution in a concentration that is vital to life.

The results for two of the practitioners and the hand-held dynamometer were exactly equal to random chance statistics. The

---

[clxiv] A dynamometer is a hand-held device that measures hand strength.

other had almost no variation from random chance.[clxv] The study also did a review of the literature on AK, and the study concluded the following:

> *The research published by the Applied Kinesiology field itself is not to be relied upon, and in the experimental studies that do meet accepted standards of science, Applied Kinesiology has **not** demonstrated that it is **a useful or reliable diagnostic tool** upon which health decisions can be based.*[66]

Another double-blind study was conducted by the ALTA Foundation for Sports Medicine Research in 1988, and also concluded this approach was *no more useful than random guessing.*[67] In 2005, yet another double-blind study concluded, *There is little or no scientific rationale for these methods. Results are not reproducible when subject to rigorous testing and do not correlate with clinical evidence of allergy.*[68]

Although clinical studies show that the results from AK are no better than random chance, anecdotal evidence is often compelling among those who use it. This dichotomy strongly suggests a spiritual source behind any results achieved.

4. Does the method used for testing or treatment ever occur through a surrogate, the phone, or by a machine that has not been scientifically proven to consistently achieve results?

Much insight into someone's health can be gleaned through conversation and physical examination. However, if a practitioner claims to be able to definitively test and know what illness or allergy exists over the phone or by testing the energy of one person through another (surrogate), beware. Because these things are not scientifically possible, the only explanations for such "results" are either chance based or demonically based, neither of which are likely to provide

---

[clxv] For those with a statistical background- the p-value was .18.

viable health solutions. The idea of a transference of energy (electric frequencies) is false, whereas the transference of spiritual power is real.

5. Is mysterious gifting required to perform the alternative practice or does the presence of certain people interfere with the effectiveness of the diagnoses or treatment? (i.e. a spouse must leave the room)

The physical explanation of how muscle testing works indicates that anyone should be capable of performing it, however; that is not the case. Many Christians cannot. My husband could test me but no one else. Furthermore, like with myself and my son, some people become remarkably "gifted" at it. Such oddities are readily explained in the spirit realm but not in the physical realm.

I have also been told by numerous Christians that their spouse was told to leave the room because their "energy" interfered with the ability to perform the test or treatment. This is easily explained by the Holy Spirit's presence rather than "energy." Furthermore, God placed the husband as the spiritual head of the home--the protector and responsible party for the family's spiritual well-being. Be particularly wary if his presence interferes with the efficacy of an alternative practice.

6. Are the methods consistent with historically Satanic practices or chance?

The Bible warns Christians to be aware of the Enemy's schemes.[clxvi] Satan's tactics change in appearance throughout time, but they follow recognizable patterns or characteristics. Paul warns that *the coming of the lawless one will be in accordance with the work of Satan displayed in all kinds of counterfeit miracles, signs and*

[clxvi] 2 Corinthians 2:11

wonders, and in every sort of evil that deceives.[clxvii] What might such counterfeit miracles look like?

From the story of Job, we know that the devil can physically harm an individual. It stands to reason, therefore, that specific symptoms caused by Satan's forces might be remedied in one of two ways: Either God orders Satan to back-off or Satan does it of his own accord. Think of it as the removal of a splinter from your hand. The hand is made better, not because of a miracle but because of the splinter's sudden absence.

In the "healing" of my thyroid, it is a reasonable possibility that, similar to Job's case of boils, Satan had been the cause of my trouble all along, and the only action necessary to affect my "healing" was to remove whatever he was doing to suppress my thyroid. Doing so at the moment of my first AK treatment created a perception that AK had healed me.

Paul also warns that *Satan himself masquerades as an angel of light. It is not surprising, then, if his servants also masquerade as servants of righteousness.*[clxviii] Over and over again, people tell me that they became ensnared with alternative practices because a Christian did it. If Satan can convince a servant of righteousness to become involved through counterfeit miracles, then he can effectively infiltrate the Christian camp.

Another consistent trait of Satan's power to affect people physically is through muscle strength or weakness.[clxix] As I said before, I became uniquely "gifted" at muscle testing. I could make a muscular man's arm go as weak as a baby's arm with the slightest downward pressure while he held one substance, even though he was easily able to stay strong while holding another. In fact, I cannot count the number of times I did this for the first time to an individual, usually a man, where a look of utter shock immediately followed their weakness, along with

---

[clxvii] 2 Thessalonians 2:9-10
[clxviii] 2 Corinthians 11:14-15
[clxix] Biblical examples of this include Mark 5:1-3, Mark 9:22.

the statement, "Wait! Do that again!" He would then visibly strain for all he was worth to keep me from again gently pushing his arm down. Accounting for this muscle weakness is critical.

Obviously, since I exist in the physical world without line-of-sight into the spiritual realm that demons inhabit, the following explanation will be just a theory, but it seems to fit the phenomena I personally experienced during my era of muscle testing: During muscle testing, "answers" to questions are revealed in a binary format, meaning that for every question asked, the muscle will give a yes or no (true or false) response. The muscle gives these binary responses by either being strong or weak in response to the question asked of the subject.

When the muscle weakens during testing, there is no odd sensation, warning the person that his/her muscle has weakened. Nor is there any sort of sense that someone in addition to the tester is exerting a force on the arm. There is only the sense that although the brain is sending signals to apply strength, those signals do not seem to reach the muscle in full force, and therefore the muscle does not respond as it should to the will of the tested subject. It is as if something has hijacked the passage of electrical signals between brain and muscle.

The similarities between the Ouija board and muscle testing are striking. Like with muscle testing, the user of a Ouija Board must first ask a question. A person, sitting at a Ouija Board with fingertips lightly touching the pointer does not detect the subtle variations in electrical signals traveling to the muscles that maintain the arms' position over the board. That person only knows or senses that without him/her willing it to do so, the marker begins to move, spelling out messages. Similar to muscle testing, some encounter nothing remarkable during an attempt to use the board; others report receiving disturbingly accurate information. I believe that muscle testing uses the human body as a Ouija Board.

7. Do the practices produce "bondage" in people?

Satan desires to ensnare people and bring them into his bondage. Beware of any alternative practice that produces an ever-increasing need for itself. Before I became involved with muscle testing, I used acupuncture for a number of months. It was remarkable how much improvement came immediately from the treatments but how short lived the relief was. It was like a drug that kept me going back over and over again for relief. This formation of dependence is bondage and an important trait to notice.

8. Do the explanations for how it works use any of the following buzzwords: energy, quantum physics, chi, chakras, the subconscious, inner child, tapping, talk of the body as though it is a separate entity-- "the body knows how to fix itself, the body doesn't lie," frequency, etc.?

Just as any field has a "lingo" that goes with it, so too does energy medicine. That wording can clue one in to recognize areas of concern. When trying to determine the validity of a particular practice, machine, therapy, or substance, notice whether certain buzzwords are used in its explanation, and if those words are frequently associated with distinctly demonic practices like muscle testing.

9. Anything that uses muscle testing in any form is divination and, therefore, forbidden for the Christian.

Numerous examples abound of substances or modalities that might or might not be intrinsically demonic but are made so by adding muscle testing to their practice. An association with AK should not be discounted. Additionally, simply asking a practitioner who uses muscle testing not to muscle test you is not advisable either. Many experienced in muscle testing do not need to make physical contact with the patient but divine the answers automatically. Such demonic empowerment will likely impact the practitioner's recommendations without your knowing it. Lastly, other forms of divination (i.e., pendulums, medical mediums) in combination with a health practice are forbidden by God.

For more information on why I am convinced that AK is divination, check out my audio lesson, "11 Reasons Muscle Testing Is Divination." https://youtu.be/Bs4tg8sJUXg.

10. Over time, does the general progression of symptoms worsen, even though there may be individual improvements? Are the symptoms that develop strange, include suicidal thoughts, or is there great fighting and strife in your home?

Through the hearing of stories from hundreds of individuals before and after repenting from involvement with energy medicine, I have noticed that a hallmark of demonically based symptoms is a suddenness of onset combined with an intensity that cannot be accounted for through normal physical responses. I have also noticed that symptoms often take on an unusual nature for which traditional medicine finds no explanation. Unexplained weakness is common, as well as neurological symptoms or extreme vertigo that cannot be explained. Extreme sensitivities to electricity and mold are commonplace in those who get involved with divination-based health practices. Practitioners frequently diagnose Lyme Disease, parasites, mold toxicity, and thyroid conditions even though standard testing (if it is even done) shows no such condition.

For some of those particular disorders, online information abounds promoting beliefs in the inadequacies of standard testing making a diagnosis that contradicts traditional test results seem believable. Satan can easily hide his torments in this way and distract people through endless "treatments" that have nothing to do with the true source of suffering. If demons are causing the symptoms in the first place, Satan has full control over when and to what degree the symptoms will exhibit. All he has to do is back off a torment that he controls in coordination with a test or treatment that he also controls in order to string someone along by giving them some "good" days.

Because Satan's goal is to destroy, pay particular attention to the presence of suicidal thoughts or debilitating fear/anxiety that develop following its use. I personally know of two individuals who committed suicide following their use of energy medicine. Another common problem not to ignore is unusual levels of strife in the home that begin or escalate after involvement with a particular health practice.

Last, take notice if a reaction to a supplement, remedy, or treatment brings immediate and significant reactions, good or bad. That is not to say that every immediate or significant reaction indicates demonic power is producing it—a severe, true allergy could also be the cause. However, if the significant reaction is atypical to accepted medical symptoms, then questions should be asked. For example, if one has seasonal allergies, the expected symptoms include sinus problems, sneezing, watery eyes, headache, and perhaps a fever. What is not expected is collapsing because of muscle weakness, stomach cramping, hallucinations, depression, unusual pain, severe anxiety, tantrums, and so on. Be careful of concluding that bizarre symptoms really are a normal reaction based on the experiences of others who also participate in energy-based health modalities or have occult ties. They could very well be deceived.

Alternative practitioners and testimonials online are quick to dismiss the ever-increasing "bad days" as being a Jarisch-Herxheimer Reaction (JHR), otherwise known as a *Herx* reaction. A true JHR is caused by the immune system reacting to the rapid die-off of harmful spirochete bacteria in response to antibiotics.[clxx] Symptoms include chills, fever, skin rashes, hypertension, myalgia, and various organ malfunctions. It typically resolves in 24 hours.[69] Alternative health practitioners often wrongly blame JHR for strong and lasting reactions in detoxifying patients to reassure their patients that the suffering indicates the therapy is working.

[clxx] Spirochetal infections include syphilis, Lyme disease, leptospirosis, and relapsing fever.

Many years ago, when I was endlessly taking supplements in an attempt to detoxify from numerous things, I was miserable day in and day out. This went on for many months without noticeable improvement, but I was assured by the practitioner and online research that this was normal. I have spoken to many who have experienced the same for months and years on end as they have sought to detoxify. They press on believing the symptoms indicate good is being accomplished even though they feel terrible. This constant state of misery is not a JHR. What truly causes the symptoms, I do not know for sure. It may be that the supplements being taken are poisoning the individual or it may be demonic torment. If this is you, I urge you to prayerfully reconsider the path you are pursuing.

11. Have you developed symptoms characterized as Lyme Disease, EMF or mold sensitivity, heavy metal poisoning, parasites, dizziness, or brain fog but have not, through traditionally accepted testing, been shown to have these conditions?

I have observed that there are a handful of likely "diagnoses" made through alternative practices. Although I cannot see or hear the spirit world, when one has had as many conversations as I have had with those coming out of energy medicine, a malicious, strategic pattern seems to emerge in the frequent diagnoses of a handful of illnesses. Practitioners frequently diagnose Lyme Disease, parasites, mold toxicity, and thyroid conditions even though standard testing (if it is even done) shows no such condition. Each of these symptoms or conditions can be real conditions.

However, the alternative medicine realm strongly promotes the hypothesis that traditional testing frequently fails to diagnose these conditions. Whether or not the traditional diagnostics for these conditions are unreliable, these are illnesses that are easily counterfeited. By calling into question traditional testing, the door is opened to assumptions and unreliable forms of testing. I have no desire to debate whether the claims about traditional testing are true. I merely wish to point out that the devil is in the counterfeit business and that these symptoms and conditions are easily counterfeited and remarkably prevalent in those who frequently use energy-based practices. This handful of conditions are easily mimicked by demonic torment and therefore controlled or escalated according to the devil's desire. Satan can easily hide his torments in this way and distract people through endless "treatments" that have nothing to do with the true source of suffering.

If you are seeking discernment regarding a particular treatment, practice, practitioner, etc., and find that these questionable symptoms and assumed diagnoses have been made, I would urge you to pause for a time of seeking the wisdom God promises to those who ask.

Modern Witchcraft

When I picture a witchdoctor, I envision a native in New Guinea with a bone through his nose and only a loin cloth to cover his flesh. In the missionary stories of my youth, such people gave potions to the tribal people that were concocted by interacting with the spirit world. I have no doubt that no "civilized" Christian would knowingly touch such a remedy with a ten-foot pole, and yet, without their knowledge, many are doing exactly that.

If the power to muscle test is indeed the result of divination, then taking any substance that is arrived at by such methods is witchcraft or sorcery. The substances themselves may or may not be helpful, but when they are chosen under demonic influence, taking them is to participate with demons. Not only is this dangerous; it is forbidden in the Bible. Attempting to attach God's holy name to such practices by praying over the treatment or remedy is to misuse His name. Paul explains the faulty logic of trying to follow God while participating with demons in 1 Corinthians 10:18-22.

Consider the people of Israel: Do not those who eat the sacrifices participate in the altar? Do I mean then that food sacrificed to an idol is anything, or that an idol is anything? No, but the sacrifices of pagans are offered to demons, not to God, and I do not want you to be participants with demons. You cannot drink the cup of the Lord and the cup of demons too; you cannot have a part in both the Lord's table and the table of demons. Are we trying to arouse the Lord's jealousy?

Essential oils are popular for treating a myriad of symptoms and conditions. Many of the combination oils have been derived from the use of AK, and the companies make no attempt to hide this fact. A simple search on muscle testing and essential oils will reveal countless "how to" videos and articles reporting the ease of creating your own combination oils through muscle testing. This is witchcraft, make no mistake.

The most prevalent use of witchcraft today occurs with homeopathy. The laborious process of dilutions and shakings in the formation of these "remedies" is done to create a spiritual remedy. (I write about homeopathy in great detail and with extensive research in *Ouija Medicine—The Dark Side of Energy Medicine*.)

Repenting & Rebuking Evil Spirits

If you have ever participated in demonic alternative practices, I urge you to repent today. Doing so brings restoration and freedom! For more detail on how to go about this and special considerations, see Appendix G.

If you unknowingly became involved with evil practices, please do not despair. Confess your sin. God's forgiveness is complete. The blood of Jesus cleanses from all sin and covers your guilt. Draw near to your Lord and Savior afresh, knowing that, just as God forgave the patriarchs of the Bible, King David, Paul, Peter, and even me, so also will God forgive you. He will allow you to be set free from the snare of the devil and to find true, complete, and lasting healing through God.

Biblical Principle: *Satan uses deception to ensnare Christians through demonically based health practices.*

Call to Action: *If you have, at any time and in any way, been a participant in demonic health practices, repent fully today and follow the biblical model described in Appendix G to rebuke any evil spirits that may be influencing you or your family.*

CHAPTER 18

Food Is NOT the Enemy

Nutrition In the Bible

And everything God created is good, and nothing is to be rejected if it is received with thanksgiving, because it is consecrated by the word of God and prayer. 1 Timothy 4:4-5

The diet recommendations of nutrition "experts" seem to change with dizzying speed as the results of each study challenges the previous. Take for example the low-fat craze that began in the '70s. "Experts" proclaimed to a trusting public that fat makes people fat and causes heart problems by clogging the arteries, both of which seemed logical.

Food manufacturers, responding to consequential market changes, greatly altered the makeup of food products to replace the then villainized cholesterol and fats with polyunsaturated oils and sugar. People replaced whole milk with skim and butter with margarine. Restaurants began frying foods with vegetable oils instead of the highly saturated fat oils of the past. Since removing fat also removes satisfying flavor, refined sugars filled in to more than compensate for the loss. Sugar consumption skyrocketed. Two hundred years ago the average American consumed only 2 pounds per year. By 1970,

American sugar intake had risen to 123 pounds per year and still continues to rise. Consumption currently runs at a staggering 150-170 pounds a year.[70]

With American willingness to embrace the low-fat craze of the last several decades, one would hope to find a trimmer nation, largely free of heart disease. Instead, obesity, diabetes, and heart disease have multiplied exponentially. According to Aaron E. Carroll, Professor of pediatrics at Indiana University School of Medicine and blog writer for *The New York Times*, it turns out the "experts" had based their advice on misconstrued findings while ignoring others that painted a very different picture.[71]

Thanks to the results of several studies done in the last few years, the proponents of the low-fat diet are now "eating humble pie." The Prospective Urban Rural Epidemiology (PURE) study followed the dietary intake of 135,335 individuals aged 35–70 years from 18 countries throughout the world for an average of 7 years. Their findings include the following:

> *Total fat and saturated and unsaturated fats were not significantly associated with risk of myocardial infarction or cardiovascular disease mortality. Higher saturated fat intake was associated with lower risk of stroke. In our replacement analyses, the strongest association on total mortality was observed when carbohydrate was replaced with polyunsaturated fatty acids.*[72]

What? Besides discovering that fat does not increase the risk of heart disease and death from heart disease, the study also found that consuming more saturated fats appears to lower the risk of stroke! Furthermore, the shift to polyunsaturated oils at the recommendation of the "trusted experts" showed the strongest link to death of any fat.

Other examples of nutritional whiplash include the demonization of eggs and salt, claims which recent studies indicate were also in error. For example, a study completed in 2016 involving 1,032 men ages 42-69 concluded that

Egg or cholesterol intakes are not associated with increased risk of coronary artery disease, even in those who are genetically predisposed to experience a stronger effect of dietary cholesterol on blood cholesterol.[73]

Even salt moved closer to vindication as the results emerged from a 2008 study measuring hospital readmissions for cardiac patients who adhered to either a low sodium or normal sodium diet following discharge. The surprising results not only revealed that a normal sodium diet greatly decreased the return visits to the hospital by people with heart disease but that depletion in sodium from a low sodium diet *has detrimental renal and neurohormonal effects.*[74]

An article in *Clinical Science* also reported the findings from eight clinical trials involving 7,200 individuals that looked at the health impact of lowering sodium intake. *None of the trials, including ones involving people with both normal and high blood pressure, showed a reduction in all-cause mortality.*[75] So, after years of doctors advising their patients to toss the salt shakers in the trash, we learn that moderate salt use keeps the kidneys and neurotransmitters optimal and can protect from many causes of death. Wow!

The shifting sands of nutritional research and dietary recommendations bring much confusion and uncertainty to any who wish to make informed decisions about what they should eat. In spite of being burned by faulty science in the past, the general public seems to have learned little. The current nutritional trends include strong recommendations to eat low carb instead of low-fat, to avoid red meat, go organic, eat a Mediterranean diet, drink coffee, and eat chocolate, just to name a few. The list of evils to avoid seems endless and includes GMO's, gluten, pesticides, preservatives, and sugar, just to name a few. The abundance of information online about the hazards of failing to jump on the latest bandwagon has produced a level of fear in the general public that borders on paranoia.

Misinterpreting Scriptures on Nutrition

Sadly, in order to make a case for this or that advice, Christians have added to the nutritional confusion by isolating out single Bible verses or advocating diets that were commonplace in the Bible only at a particular time or region. For example, the Mediterranean diet has gained current popularity among many Christians who teach that it is THE God-ordained diet. After all, olives were abundant in Israel, and Jesus multiplied the fish. They ignore the detail that the Savior did the same with gluten-laden barley loaves.

The Bible gives much instruction about food, but it also tells of varied diets of the Bible characters as part of the narrative of their lives. These details are generally meant to be descriptive, not prescriptive. To conclude that the diet of a particular Bible character is God's will for all of mankind is bad theology.

Ezekiel bread is my personal favorite example of nutritional advice based on bad interpretation of Scripture. In Ezekiel 4:9, God gave the prophet Ezekiel a recipe for bread made of sprouted grains and beans that he was to eat for forty days to represent the coming of forty years of siege on Jerusalem. A quick glance at the context reveals that this bread was intended to communicate God's reproach. To highlight His people's uncleanness and the removal of God's blessing, the bread was to be baked on human excrement. I fail to see how a positive conclusion can be established from this passage that we should eat such bread.

Another faulty conclusion on dietary matters from Scripture comes from the instance of Daniel and his friends consuming only vegetables and water when first brought to Babylon as captives. The young men did so out of a desire to obey God, whose dietary laws declared some of the king's food "unclean." Yes, God did indeed bless them with intelligence, strength, vitality, and wisdom while on the diet.[clxxi] However, at some point during Daniel's life in Babylon, we know that

---

[clxxi] Daniel 1

he changed to a diet that included meat and wine because Daniel 10:3 speaks of him fasting from such foods. Therefore, concluding that a long-term vegetarian diet is healthy or God-ordained is to ignore countless passages that speak of eating meat.

In reading the stories of the Bible, we can see great variety over time in the way people ate and in what God commanded. To truly understand a biblical perspective on nutrition, we must look at the big picture in Scripture--the heart of God. God is good and loves to bless His people.

Tracing "God's Diet" Through the Bible

If you want to discover the central idea behind the abundance of Scriptural instruction on food, understand this: **All food is good and meant by God to be a satisfying blessing.** At different periods in the Bible, God changed the specific instructions to His people about what should be eaten, but without exception, food was meant to bless and satisfy.

At creation, God instructed Adam to enjoy eating every fruit and seed-bearing plant, with the caveat that two certain trees were off-limits.[clxxii] God seemed to take pride in the fact that what He offered to Adam and Eve was "good." Genesis 2:9 said, *The LORD God made all kinds of trees grow out of the ground—trees that were pleasing to the eye and good for food.* Because sin and death had not yet entered creation, man could not kill the animals for food.

Jumping ahead to the time immediately following the world-wide flood, God instructed Noah that he could then eat anything he desired. *Everything that lives and moves about will be food for you. Just as I gave you the green plants, I now give you everything.*[clxxiii] This time

---

[clxxii] Genesis 1:29-30 & 2:8-9, 16
[clxxiii] Genesis 9:3

the only restriction that is given was not to eat meat that had its *lifeblood still in it.*[clxxiv]

The next direct biblical instruction on food came with the institution of the lengthy, dietary laws God gave through Moses in Leviticus 11. In those laws, God detailed which foods, from birds to fish to livestock, were "clean." Those laws were meant to set God's people apart from the surrounding nations and to preserve them. Therefore, some Christians conclude that, although the New Testament freed God's children from the law, the dietary laws should still be followed because they reflect what God knows is best for optimal health.

Although those laws seemed restrictive, the heart of God still shone through. God desired to bless and satisfy His people through food. Deuteronomy 8 provides one of many examples that express that desire.

> *For the Lord your God is bringing you into a good land ...a land with wheat and barley, vines and fig trees, pomegranates, olive oil and honey; a land where bread will not be scarce and you will lack nothing...When you have eaten and are satisfied, praise the Lord your God for the good land he has given you. Be careful that you do not forget the Lord your God, failing to observe his commands, his laws and his decrees that I am giving you this day.*

From this point forward in the Old Testament, God repeatedly stated His desire to bless and satisfy His people through food, if they would only follow Him. Every food group was included in list after list throughout the OT, but three items, in particular, were singled out as the definitive sign of God's blessing--grain (bread), wine, and oil. The Bible repeatedly states that the removal of the blessing of those foods comes when His people walk in sin. As previously mentioned, the recipe for Ezekiel bread is a blatant example of this, but here are a just

---

[clxxiv] Genesis 9:4

a few more of the many passages that express the same idea, as well as highlighting the three primary dietary blessings--grain (bread), wine, and oil.

- *So if you faithfully obey the commands I am giving you today then I will send rain on your land in its season so that you may gather in your grain, new wine and olive oil. I will provide grass in the fields for your cattle, and you will eat and be satisfied.* (Deuteronomy 11:13-15)

- *He waters the mountains from his upper chambers; the land is satisfied by the fruit of his work. He makes grass grow for the cattle, and plants for people to cultivate—bringing forth food from the earth: wine that gladdens human hearts, oil to make their faces shine, and bread that sustains their hearts.* (Psalm 104:13-15)

- *The Lord their God will save his people on that day as a shepherd saves his flock. They will sparkle in his land like jewels in a crown. How attractive and beautiful they will be! Grain will make the young men thrive, and new wine the young women.* (Zechariah 9:16-17)

- *She has not acknowledged that I was the one who gave her the grain, the new wine and oil, who lavished on her the silver and gold—which they used for Baal. "Therefore I will take away my grain when it ripens, and my new wine when it is ready. "In that day I will respond,"...declares the Lord—"I will respond to the skies, and they will respond to the earth; and the earth will respond to the grain, the new wine and the olive oil.* (Hosea 2:8-10, 21-22)

- *The eyes of all look to you, and you give them their food at the proper time. You open your hand and satisfy the desires of every living thing.* (Psalm 145:15-16)

The New Testament teaching on food continued in the same vein but became even more forthright. In Acts 10, we learn that the apostle

Peter had a vision while taking an afternoon nap. Three times creatures of all kinds, including those that God had previously declared unclean through Moses, were lowered in a canopy from heaven.

A voice from heaven said, Get up, Peter. Kill and eat.

Peter responded with indignation. Surely not, Lord! I have never eaten anything impure or unclean.

The voice replied, Do not call anything impure that God has made clean.[clxxv]

From the story, we learn that God intended for the dream to announce, not only God's acceptance of all food but also all people. As the Creator of all things, God alone has the power and privilege to make something or someone clean.

Everything Is Good

In our continuing progression through biblical teachings on food, we come to a definitive passage that foretells of the wrong teaching that the end times will bring to pass. 1 Timothy 4:1-5 says,

The Spirit clearly says that in later times some will abandon the faith and follow deceiving spirits and things taught by demons. Such teachings come through hypocritical liars, whose consciences have been seared as with a hot iron. They forbid people to marry and order them to abstain from certain foods, which God created to be received with thanksgiving by those who believe and who know the truth. For everything God created is good, and nothing is to be rejected if it is received with thanksgiving, because it is consecrated by the word of God and prayer.

[clxxv] Acts 10:13-15

Currently, how many foods have we been told "to abstain" from, and how many of those have you personally chosen to "reject"--gluten, wheat, dairy of any kind, red meat or meat of any kind, natural sugars, certain sweet vegetables or fruits, things containing natural fat (i.e., eggs, butter, and whole milk), or wine? God says that they are all "good" and should be received with thanksgiving!

I know the arguments that will arise in people's minds upon reading that conclusion. "But I'm lactose intolerant!" Or, "I've developed leaky gut syndrome from gluten and, therefore, I feel bad if I don't abstain from all gluten." Or, "our food supply has become tainted by pesticides and GMO's and the soil is so depleted that food no longer provides the nutrition needed anyway. Supplements are the way to go." Or, "Eating meat is cruel to animals; so, I will not eat any animal products!" On and on the list of culturally popular beliefs go, just as Paul warned it would.

The ongoing nutritional assertions of science continue to stoke fear, but as we have seen by looking at history, these assertions change with the wind. What never changes is the heart of God. His Word is clear. The LORD desires to satisfy those who walk with Him with the food He created. While speaking of the many "benefits" God gives to His children, King David says, *who satisfies your <u>mouth</u> with good things so that your youth is renewed like the eagle's* (Psalm 103:4 KJV). Unfortunately, a poor translation of the Hebrew word "mouth" to "desires," is made in other Bible versions which waters down the intended and crystal-clear meaning. God not only wishes to satisfy His children's mouths with good food, but it is by that very food that renewal takes place.

Carbohydrates in the Bible

Bread remains one of the most satisfying foods throughout time; yet, it has recently come under comprehensive attack. This source of carbohydrates stands alone in Scripture as the single most prominent

food representing God's blessing.   Jesus is the "bread of life."[clxxvi]
Biblical writers speak of bread around three hundred times throughout
Scripture.   God fed the Israelites on bread from heaven for forty years.
When people needed their strength renewed, it was bread that was
given.[clxxvii]   God instituted an annual, seven-day festival where the
people ate only bread.[clxxviii]   The priests placed loaves of unleavened
bread before the LORD daily.[clxxix]   Many of the sacrifices the Israelites
offered included bread.[clxxx]   Psalm 104:15 claims that bread *sustains
the heart*.   Proverbs 30:8 and the Lord's prayer reference *daily bread.*

     When God removes His blessing, the Bible singles out the absence
of satisfying bread as the evidence.[clxxxi]   Now some might have us
believe that this bread of blessing was made with unusual grains such
as spelt, amaranth, and millet rather than wheat or barley.   However,
spelt makes an appearance in the Bible only three times, one of which
is in the Ezekiel 4:9 bread, as does millet.   In contrast, the now
demonized, gluten-rich wheat appears forty-six times and always as an
indicator of God's great blessing.[clxxxii]   As the poor man's grain of
choice, barley (also high in gluten) came close behind that of wheat as
a sign of God's blessing and appears thirty-five times in Scripture.

     With all of this biblical talk of bread and grain, you might wonder
about the soundness of current low-carb recommendations.   Whether or
not the science holds in coming decades or suffers a similar fate as the
low-fat trend, I cannot say.   I can, however, say that biblically
speaking, no support for such thinking exists.

     In light of all of this, I have two theories as to why so many people
get sick when they eat gluten or other particular foods.   First, their
bodies may be responding to a fear of those foods because of the

---

clxxvi John 6:35, 48, & 51
clxxvii i.e., Judges 8:5, 1 Sam.21:3, 1 Kin.17:6, 11-12, 19:6, 2 Kin.4:42
clxxviii Exodus 23:15
clxxix Exodus 40:23, Leviticus 24:8
clxxx Leviticus 23:18
clxxxi Amos 4:6, 2 Cor.9:10
clxxxii i.e., Deut.8:8

abundant hype about their dangers. I experienced this and will discuss a recommendation for how to overcome this problem at the end of the chapter. Second, perhaps God has removed His blessing on you by making you unable to digest the elements representing His blessing because of some sin in your life. This removal of blessing is not intended by your loving Savior to be permanent but to alert you to your sin that you might repent and again enjoy the Lord's blessing.

The supposed biblical support of the Mediterranean diet, with its plant-based emphasis and elimination of dairy and red meat, also seems strangely lacking. Instead, a varied diet with a variety of livestock meats, fruits and vegetables, dairy, wine, and the grains wheat and barley in abundance take center stage.[clxxxiii] Lists of foods abound in the biblical stories, and carbohydrates top the lists with grains, cakes of figs and raisins, honey, and wine.[clxxxiv] Oddly enough, fish remains absent from the Old Testament food lists. Fish makes more of an appearance in the Gospels because many of the stories occur near the Sea of Galilee where fishing was a way of life.

God's Perfect Design for Food

About a decade ago, someone told me about the book <u>Nourishing Traditions,</u> and I began to devour its contents with fascination. With extensive research citations, popular author and speaker Sally Fallon and co-author, Mary G. Enig, Ph.D., an expert of international renown in the field of chemistry, describe a complex world I once knew nothing about: the incredible complexity of how the body absorbs and utilizes the minerals and nutrients that food affords. Each dietary component impacts another in a complex cascade. Like the old-style Christmas tree lights where if one bulb burnt out, the whole string failed to light, so also is nutritional absorption. If one of the parts of the nutritional chain is missing or there is too much or too little, the entire process is affected.

[clxxxiii] i.e., 2 Sam.17:28-29, 1 Chron.12:40, 2 Chron.31:5-6, Joel 1
[clxxxiv] i.e., 2 Sam. 6:19 & 16:1,

Even though nothing in *Nourishing Traditions* speaks of a biblical perspective on nutrition, I noticed clearly in its contents evidence that the Creator, infinite in knowledge and understanding, designed food for the human body. Although this topic is endless and science has only touched the surface of understanding the seemingly endless intricacies of food absorption, I would like to quote a number of examples from Fallon and Enig:

- *Protein cannot be adequately utilized without dietary fats. That is why protein and fats occur together in eggs, milk, fish, and meats.*[76]

- *Digestion of refined carbohydrates call on the body's own store of vitamins, minerals and enzymes for proper metabolization. When B vitamins are absent, for example, the breakdown of carbohydrates cannot take place, yet most B vitamins are removed during the refining process* (of grains).[77]

- *Heat alters milk's amino acids lysine and tyrosine, making the whole complex of proteins less available...pasteurization destroys all the enzymes in milk. These enzymes* (such as lactase) *help the body assimilate all bodybuilding factors, including calcium...Lipase in raw milk helps the body digest and utilize butterfat.*[78]

- Vitamin A *is a catalyst on which innumerable biochemical processes depend...neither protein, minerals nor water-soluble vitamins can be utilized by the body without vitamin A from animal sources...Carotenes are converted to vitamin A in the upper intestine...but studies have shown that our bodies cannot convert carotenes into vitamin A without the presence of fat in the diet. Proper iodine utilization requires sufficient levels of vitamin A, supplied by animal fats.*[79]

- *The second most abundant mineral in the body, phosphorus is needed for bone growth, kidney function, and cell growth...Phosphorus is found in many foods, but in order to be properly utilized, it must be in proper balance with magnesium and calcium in the blood.*[80]

Putting the Biblical Principle in Action

God intricately designed the human body to require a host of vitamins, minerals, acids, fats, proteins, enzymes, and so on, and they all work in concert with each other to perform complicated biochemical processes. Although a study of the complexities of nutrition proves fascinating, in reality, God made it very simple for humans. Everything God created is good! Rather than getting bogged down in the details of nutrition, my goal has been to give the big, unchanging picture from Scripture-- that **all food is good and meant by God to be a satisfying blessing.**

In the New Testament, God gives freedom for people to eat as they choose or how their individual conscience dictates. The only boundaries given are to avoid gluttony, drunkenness, or eating habits that might lead others astray.

Consider, if you will, two areas of practical application. First, the claim that ALL food created by God is good and not to be rejected out of fear (where no personal and definitive medical diagnosis exists) does not extend to foods created by man. If you want a simple guide for choosing what foods and what forms of that food are "healthy," then ask one simple question--Did God make it? If the answer is "yes," then go for it regardless of what current popular opinion says. If it has been processed, refined, or preserved in unnatural ways and therefore, altered from its original state in some fashion such as with white flour, white sugar, homogenization,[clxxxv] pasteurization, hydrogenation,[clxxxvi]

[clxxxv] The process by which the fat (cream) in milk is forced through extreme pressure into extremely small particles so that it remains uniform throughout the milk. http://www.raw-milk-facts.com/homogenization_T3.html
[clxxxvi] This is the chemical treatment done to turn liquid vegetable oil into a solid by chemically treating it using hydrogen and a metal such as nickel.

chemical or extremely high heat treatments, then the label of "good" does not apply.

Although I personally watch what I eat quite carefully to make sure that the bulk of my diet comes from a wide variety of whole foods, I do not stress over the **occasional** addition of man-altered foods. Why? Because I know that more important than the food itself is the fact that God desires to bless and satisfy me through food. Sometimes a chocolate cake made with white sugar and white flour satisfies as nothing else can, so I eat it with the freedom and blessing of the Lord.

That leads me to the second application I wish to make. Fear of food that God has called good is from Satan and should be dealt with as such. Sometimes this fear emanates from knowledge gained from abundant sources on potentially detrimental foods or things related to food. Often, though, the fear comes from the negative, physical reaction (pain, digestive distress, headaches, etc.) that someone comes to associate with food. Frequently, this powerful association between food and physical discomfort is not the result of a true allergy or Celiac Disease but the plastic brain responding to fear. Neurons that wire together, fire together.

We also learned in the chapter on the heart that thoughts and emotions directly trigger the autonomic nervous system, thereby stimulating the digestive system. Therefore, negative thoughts and emotions while eating will have a tremendous impact on the body's response to food.

This was the case with me. Although I did have true allergies to a handful of foods (based on blood allergy testing), over time more and more foods made me sick. I eventually got to the place where just putting any food or liquid in my mouth would send my stomach into spasm, and then it would swell up like a balloon about to burst. It took me years to discover that I somehow needed to change the nerve pathways in my brain so that I no longer considered food to be the enemy. Since the Bible speaks of being transformed by the renewing of our minds by truth, I decided to try a particular tactic that worked beautifully.

I wrote 1 Timothy 4:4-5 on a notecard and would read it as part of my prayer of blessing before I ate anything. It says, *For everything God created is good, and nothing is to be rejected if it is received with thanksgiving, because it is consecrated by the word of God and prayer.* I would then go on to pray something like this, "Lord, thank you that this food you have given me IS good, and I trust you to make it a blessing to my body."

Over the course of that first couple of weeks of praying that passage, my physical reactions to food diminished until they largely disappeared. When they occasionally reappear, I remind myself of God's truth and make sure not to take too much notice. The brain is quick to make powerful associations, and I know that an occasional reaction to food is completely normal.

Another attitude toward food that is counter to God's Word is the rejection of a whole class of foods because of preference. Those who do so could defend their decision with Paul's words from 1 Corinthians 10:23. *I have the right to do anything.* Yet the apostle Paul responded, *but not everything is beneficial.* Rejecting green vegetables or meat because you find them gross is in contradiction to 1 Timothy 4. Often people who reject whole classes of foods replace them with something far less beneficial, like supplements, or even overtly unhealthy foods, such as soy products or processed foods. As demonstrated by the previous quotes from *Nourishing Traditions*, the body's complex biochemical processes stay optimized by components from all the various food groups. To attempt to replace food groups through supplements is, at best, educated guesswork and can easily produce imbalances that impact health.

Changing the way one thinks about food can be challenging. Can you imagine the difficulty that New Testament, Jewish believers had in overcoming their aversion to foods that had been declared "unclean" for thousands of years? However, the Jewish apostles taught the reception of all foods with thanksgiving, *because (they are) consecrated by the word of God and prayer.*[clxxxvii]   Do you struggle with a fear of or dislike for foods that keep you from enjoying the incredible variety that God created for your satisfaction and enjoyment? Let God's Word consecrate all food so that you may enjoy His blessing.

> *Come, all you who are thirsty, come to the waters; and you who have no money, come, buy and eat! Come, buy wine and milk without money and without cost. Why spend money on what is not bread, and your labor on what does not satisfy? Listen, listen to me, and eat what is good, and you will delight in the richest of fare. Give ear and come to me; listen, that you may live.* (Isaiah 55:1-3)

Biblical Principle: *All food is good and meant by God to be a satisfying blessing.*

Call to Action: *The next time you pray before eating, think about the truth from 1 Timothy 4:1-5, tell the Lord of your thankfulness that the food He has given you is good.*

If you have food sensitivities, prayerfully consider whether they might exist because of an area of sin in your life that has caused God to remove His blessing.

When you read or hear nutritional advice, ask yourself before implementing it--"How does it match up to the unchanging truth of God's Word?"

[clxxxvii] 1 Timothy 4:5

CHAPTER 19

The Sins of the Fathers--
Change Your Genetic Destiny

Knowing that you were ransomed from the futile ways inherited from your forefathers, not with perishable things such as silver or gold, but with the precious blood of Christ. 1 Peter 1:18-19

After decades of a mere shadowy understanding of DNA, the scientific community rejoiced, when, in 1953, James Watson and Francis Crick discovered the double-helix structure of DNA, which seemed to unlock the mysteries of the genetic code. "DNA is destiny," became the mantra of science, and every disease, hang-up, and weakness could now be blamed on bad genes. After all, who can resist the blueprint for all life? Your fate is sealed, or so it was thought until 2003.

A Code On Top of a Code

In 2003, Dr. Randy Jirtle astounded the scientific community with the results of a landmark study involving mice. These particular mice were made obese and distinctly yellow as a result of a specific gene called the Agouti gene. According to the conventional understanding of genetics, the offspring of these mice should always exhibit the weight and color characteristics passed down to them by their parents. However, following the implementation of an aggressive vitamin regimen, something shocking happened. The Agouti mice produced brown, skinny offspring![81] How could such a thing be? In one fell swoop, the Agouti mice study crushed the mantra that genes are destiny and set the course for a new field of study--epigenetics.

In computer speak, if genetics is the hardware, epigenetics is the software. The genetic code remains constant, but the epigenome is malleable. Although genes may provide the blueprint for life, epigenetic markers turn on or off the expression of those genes like light switches. In the case of the Agouti mice, the vitamins changed one type of epigenetic marker (DNA methylation), and voila, the Agouti gene that causes obesity and yellow fur turned off.

The almost six-foot-long DNA strand is wound like thread on spools, known as histones, in order to compactly fit into the nucleus of every living cell. The grouping of histones, known as a chromatin, has various kinds of epigenetic markers that sit on top of them, dictating whether the information within will be so tightly wound up that the information becomes unreadable or if it will be decompressed, allowing for full expression. Aptly named epigenetics (*epi* means above) this study is quite literally a code on top of a code. To use another computer analogy, because of the length of information in each DNA strand, they become zip files. The epigenetic markers resting on top of a particular file (gene) determine which ones will be unzipped and therefore, readable.

The human implications of epigenetics are endless, and new directions for research have multiplied again and again throughout the last decade. These markers are heritable but changeable. So, even though you carry the gene for a particular disease, it does not mean that your fate is set in stone. Jirtle explained it this way.

The deterministic part in our system is the DNA. That's the stable part. The free will part comes in through the software that tells that deterministic (part) *how to work. We are, in effect, a programmable computer. That's how we were made.*[82]

At conception, embryogenesis begins when the sperm joins with an egg and the union between two separate genetic and epigenetic codes occurs. Research currently indicates that through a process called reprogramming all but about 10% of the male epigenetic code and all of the female's gets erased.[83] This reprogramming means that each of the 250 types of cells to be formed in the human body can begin with a nearly blank slate of DNA markers. However, based on the presence of the few remaining markers from the father, each new cell is directed to become a heart cell or a liver cell or a nerve cell and so on until each and every cell of the new life has been created.[84] Epigenetic changes are cell-specific. The markers found in the liver may be different from those found in the heart or the brain, which explains how certain diseases impact only specific parts of the body.

Science now understands that most cancers and disease, in general, have an epigenetic basis. Max Planck, author of *Epigenetics Between the Generations: We Inherit More Than Just Genes*, writes,

Contrary to the fixed sequence of 'letters' in our DNA, epigenetic marks can also change throughout our life and in response to our environment or lifestyle. For example, smoking changes the epigenetic makeup of lung cells, eventually leading to cancer.[85]

According to Fazlul H. Sarkar, editor of Epigenetics and Cancer, *tumor dormancy is considered the last battle to cure cancer*[86] and discovering pharmaceutical or nutraceutical agents that can safely turn off the epigenetic switches that affect cancer stem cells could be the cure for which everyone has been waiting. In theory, learning how to manipulate the epigenetic markers that cause disease would cure every disease, but reality proves far more complex. Endless questions remain.

The Sins of the Fathers

Sperm not only determines the sex of the embryo, but it also contains epigenetic markers necessary for embryogenesis to rightly proceed.[87]   The importance of the father's epigenetics in the proper development of the embryo explains the past mystery as to why a number of problems have arisen from in vitro fertilization (IVF); i.e., short-term pregnancies and the sometimes shorter stature of the offspring. Because IVF frequently uses the sperm from infertile men (slow sperm or low sperm count), a less-than-optimal epigenetic code is passed on to the embryo, affecting normal development.[88]

Because embryogenesis requires the paternal epigenetic code, some of the father's other epigenetic markers also get passed down from one generation to the next.[89]   Multiple studies reveal that everything from traumatic events to the way those in the paternal lineage ate or lived shape the epigenetics contained in the father's sperm and can be passed down to future generations.[90]

On the other hand, in humans, the mother's epigenetic code, washed away at conception, appears to form afresh within hours based on the conditions present during pregnancy.[91]   Therefore, the mother's diet, health, and state of mind during pregnancy become powerful forces shaping the formation of the growing child's epigenetic code, thereby greatly affecting the future health of the offspring. (The next chapter will address the ongoing parental impact throughout childhood as a child's epigenome continues to form.)

The Bible draws frequent attention to the idea that sin and its effects pass specifically through the father's line. Evidence of the paternal epigenome's profound and multi-faceted impact on future generations is so strong that a secular, scientific abstract reviewing the last ten years of research actually begins by quoting Exodus 20:5. *For I the Lord your God am a jealous God, visiting the iniquity of the fathers on the children to the third and the fourth generation of those who hate me* (ESV).[92]   The abstract cites studies that confirm both heavy drinking and smoking produce inheritable epigenetic markers in the father's line, going back multiple generations.[93]

In surprising contrast, human studies to date indicate that similar addictive behaviors of the mother herself, not her ancestors, impact the growing child.[94] Interestingly, the epigenetic differentiation between the impact of a mother's choices during pregnancy and child-rearing versus multiple generations of the father's lifestyle choices getting passed down seems to be referenced in Psalm 109:14. *May the iniquity of his fathers be remembered before the Lord; may the sin of his mother never be blotted out.* This verse references fathers, meaning multiple generations, and their iniquity (guilt and punishment from sin)[95] being remembered. However, it speaks only of the singular mother and her sin being remembered. Epigenetic research confirms this teaching from Scripture.

Although we cannot understand the exact nature or link between the spiritual and the physical, epigenetics would appear to be the physical means God chose to implement the spiritual legacy of sin. Could this explain how all mankind inherited a sin nature through Adam? *Therefore, just as sin entered the world through one man, and death through sin, and in this way death came to all people.*[clxxxviii] Dr. Norman Geisler, PhD., author of over a hundred books and a conservative, evangelical theologian, believes the answer is yes.[96] Jesus Christ came through a virgin mother who, like us, needed a savior,[clxxxix] and yet her son, conceived by the Holy Spirit and not a man, was without sin.[cxc]

Choosing Your Own Path

Ezekiel 18 reveals God's perspective on the sins of the fathers by quoting a proverb that pictures the impact of epigenetics. *The fathers*

[clxxxviii] Romans 5:12
[clxxxix] Luke 1:46
[cxc] Matthew 1:18 & 20, 2 Corinthians 5:21

have eaten sour grapes, and the children's teeth are set on edge.[cxci]
Even though the proverb clearly describes truth, it does not give the
whole picture and so God goes on to clarify in great detail through the
prophet Ezekiel. Although the sins of the fathers might be passed
down, each new generation has the opportunity to wipe the slate clean
by choosing not to walk according to the sins of their fathers. Even
though the passage is long, the details help us understand God's design
for epigenetics so that we might then make appropriate applications for
health.

> *Behold, all souls are mine; the soul of the father as well as the
> soul of the son is mine: the soul who sins shall die. "If a man is
> righteous and does what is just and right—walks in my statutes,
> and keeps my rules by acting faithfully—he is righteous; he shall
> surely live, declares the Lord God.*
>
> *If he fathers a son who is violent, a shedder of blood, who does
> any of these things (though he himself did none of these things),
> He shall not live. He has done all these abominations; he shall
> surely die; his blood shall be upon himself.*
>
> *Now suppose this man fathers a son who sees all the sins that his
> father has done; he sees, and does not do likewise: he shall not
> die for his father's iniquity; he shall surely live. As for his father,
> because he practiced extortion, robbed his brother, and did what
> is not good among his people, behold, he shall die for his
> iniquity.*
>
> *Yet you say, 'Why should not the son suffer for the iniquity of
> the father?' When the son has done what is just and right, and
> has been careful to observe all my statutes, he shall surely live.
> The soul who sins shall die. The son shall not suffer for the
> iniquity of the father, nor the father suffer for the iniquity of the
> son. The righteousness of the righteous shall be upon himself,
> and the wickedness of the wicked shall be upon himself.*

[cxci] Ezekiel 18:2 ESV

Therefore I will judge you, O house of Israel, every one according to his ways, declares the Lord God. Repent and turn from all your transgressions, lest iniquity be your ruin. Cast away from you all the transgressions that you have committed, and make yourselves a new heart and a new spirit! Why will you die, O house of Israel? For I have no pleasure in the death of anyone, declares the Lord God; so turn, and live.[cxcii]

Yes, through epigenetics the Creator put in place a physical means by which the punishment for the sins of the fathers might potentially be felt by future generations. This truth should bring great pause to all people as they consider that their sinful choices not only affect them but their children, grandchildren, and great-grandchildren.

However, God, in His infinite mercy, also put in place the epigenetic reality that inherited markers can be changed based on the current choices of the individual. Neither DNA nor epigenetics is destiny! According to Scripture, no one is cursed by God because of his or her ancestors' sinful ways. Again, science only has a vague understanding of the factors that can turn off the expression of genetics. The interworking of the spiritual impacting the physical may be the link science is missing.

In the Old Testament, one also finds instances of the Israelites confessing the sins of their fathers, as well as their own.[cxciii] Some might conclude from these Old Testament teachings and practices that it is necessary for Christians to discover the sins of their fathers so that those sins can be confessed, thereby removing God's punishment for sin in the present. However, the New Testament authors never speak of this practice, and understanding the reason is a game-changer. The reason rests in understanding a believer's new life in Christ.

New Life in Christ

[cxcii] Ezekiel 18:4-20, 30-32
[cxciii] Leviticus 26:40, Nehemiah 9:1-3

Sinless Jesus took on the flesh of a man through the line of David, and yet because He was born of a woman and the Holy Spirit, He did not inherit the sin nature of Adam. Remember, the mother's former epigenetic code is washed away at conception. As a result, He alone, as the spotless lamb of God, could take on the punishment for sin in our stead. By sanctifying the flesh through His physical suffering and death and being raised to new life, He offers to all the hope of new life in Him.

1 Corinthians 15:45-49 speaks of our inheritance from Adam being replaced by the last Adam, Christ.

> *So it is written: "The first man Adam became a living being"; the last Adam, a life-giving spirit. The spiritual did not come first, but the natural, and after that the spiritual. The first man was of the dust of the earth; the second man is of heaven.*

> *As was the earthly man, so are those who are of the earth; and as is the heavenly man, so also are those who are of heaven. And just as we have borne the image of the earthly man, so shall we bear the image of the heavenly man.*

Through faith in Jesus, an individual who was originally born in the image of the earthly man is suddenly "born again" to bear the image of the heavenly man. Thus, all believers belong to *the church of the firstborn*, whose names are written in heaven.[cxciv] What does this new birth mean exactly? According to 2 Corinthians 5:17, *If anyone is in Christ he is a new creation, the old has gone, the new has come*.

Although the Bible clearly teaches the doctrine of new life in Christ, many Christians do not understand it and generally continue to live as though the old has not been replaced by something completely new and different. But what if epigenetics is the physical means used by the Holy Spirit to bring to pass the spiritual reality spoken of in Scripture? Let us consider such a possibility.

[cxciv] Hebrews 12:22-23

Scientists know that epigenetic changes occur all the time, but they do not understand the complexity of factors that bring these changes to pass. What science has learned, though, is that significant events set in motion a myriad of physical responses that shape the epigenome and alter genetic expression. Norman Geisler reasons that regeneration through faith in Christ is a significant event, and, therefore, must produce system-wide epigenetic changes.[97]

What if the new birth spoken of in Scripture is quite literally a new birth of part or all of the epigenetic code, giving believers who walk according to the Spirit the image of the sinless Christ? Even so, the heart still contains the fleshly soul with all of its desires, and the sinful patterns of thinking from the mind still need transforming by the truth of God. However, rather than being bound by the sins of the fathers and the law of sin and death, Christians truly have become a new creation and must learn to walk accordingly in order to experience the new reality. Is that not what 1 Peter 1 explains?

> *As obedient children, do not be conformed to the passions of your former ignorance, but as he who called you is holy, you also be holy in all your conduct...knowing that you were ransomed from the futile ways inherited from your forefathers, not with perishable things such as silver or gold, but with the precious blood of Christ...*
>
> *Having purified your souls by obedience to the truth...since you have been born again, not of perishable seed but of imperishable, through the living and abiding word of God.[cxcv]*

There, we see our next biblical principle of health: **The inheritance of the fathers need not determine the health of someone who is IN Christ.**

Therefore, no need exists to confess the sins of the fathers because, IN Christ, we have literally been ransomed from their physical

---

[cxcv] 1 Peter 1:14-15, 18-19, 22-23 ESV

impact and born again with a new nature. However, according to Scripture, there is a significant caveat. The old nature still resides within us and remains turned off only so long as we remain IN Christ. We must allow the indwelling Holy Spirit to govern our minds in order to reap the benefits of life and peace.[cxcvi] Then, what is true of Christ becomes true of us.

All Things Are New

The other day I spoke with a Christian woman who described to me her life-long struggle with anxiety, and how she had found a measure of relief and control through an alternative therapy. She said that she could not imagine life without phobias and anxiousness. We all have struggles in our lives that seem to dictate our responses in life. In the next chapter, I will show how scientific research indicates that much of this stems from epigenetic markers brought about through inheritance or our own exposures.

For me, depression once characterized my days, and for most of my life, I could not have imagined anything different. However, as I described in chapter 7, when I began to take literally the teaching that I AM a new creation IN Christ, that truth became my reality through the Holy Spirit. Depression has no hold on me IN Christ. I am, quite literally, a new creation. When Satan comes knocking with a reminder that Marci gets depressed, I respond by reminding myself that that was the old Marci, and she is gone. Christ made me a new creation IN Him. I am not bound by the tendency towards depression I likely inherited genetically and then reinforced by my own experiences and patterns of thought. I have been set free in Christ for four years and counting.

Forgetting What Is Behind

Are you a believer in Jesus Christ as your Savior? If so, do you continue to live as though the old you still has the power to dictate who

---

[cxcvi] Romans 8:6

you are? It should have been replaced by the new long ago. Yes, obesity, addictions, depression, OCD, anxiety, homosexuality, inability to handle stress, and many other conditions have a link to epigenetic markers that can turn up the volume on certain genes. But (this is HUGE) you ARE a new creation IN CHRIST! Say it out loud--*I AM a NEW creation IN Christ!* Say it again and again! *The old has gone, behold, all things are made new*! (KJV).

At two periods in my life, I have personally received great benefit from counseling in order to work through traumas of the past and certainly do not wish to discourage anyone from seeking a wise, Christian counselor for such purposes. However, I have known many people who become stuck looking back. Past hurts hold their gaze. I fear that the study of genetics and epigenetics might add to that backward focus, which is certainly not my intent.

The reason we do not need to confess the sins of the fathers is that we are new in Christ. In a beautiful passage in Philippians, Paul speaks of his past, and how he considered it, and anything else besides Christ, *rubbish*. Instead, his sole focus rested on Jesus. Acknowledging his failures, though, he says,

> *Not that I have already obtained all this, or have already arrived at my goal, but I press on to take hold of that for which Christ Jesus took hold of me. Brothers and sisters, I do not consider myself yet to have taken hold of it. But one thing I do: Forgetting what is behind and straining toward what is ahead, I press on toward the goal to win the prize for which God has called me heavenward in Christ Jesus.*[cxcvii]

What need do those whom Christ has made new have to look at what is gone? We are no longer slaves to the past. We have been set free! During a discussion where Jesus compared His own Father with the sinful inheritance of the earthly fathers of the Jews, Jesus said; *Then you will know the truth, and the truth will set you free,* and *so if*

[cxcvii] Philippians 3:12-14

the Son sets you free, you will be free indeed.[cxcviii] What a glorious thing it is to be free!

I do not know, nor has science yet proven, whether physical illnesses can truly be ended by turning off the epigenetic switches that trigger a disease's onset. However, the theory that such is the case is quite strong, and the research proceeds with great fervor. Though I cannot say with certainty, it also seems likely that our heavenly Father uses epigenetics as one means to bring healing from all manner of inherited disease. The key to such changes is not a drug, though, but the Holy Spirit. The flesh brings sin and death, but the Spirit brings life and peace. Which one will you choose? Walk in new life through the Spirit!

Biblical Principle: *The inheritance of the fathers need not determine the health of someone who is IN Christ.*

Call to Action: *What remnants of the old you or past generations have you been allowing to dictate your current reality? In your mind or in writing confess them as sin to the Lord. Acknowledge to your loving Savior that you have been living as though the old you controlled your thoughts, emotions, and behavior rather than your new life in Christ.*

If you wrote the sin down, burn it as a visual reminder that God's Word says the old is gone.

Let your new mantra be, "I AM a new creation IN CHRIST. My sin of _____ is part of the old your name. The old is gone. The new has come." Repeat that mantra every time the old patterns return.

[cxcviii] John 6:32 & 36

CHAPTER 20

Epigenetics
& Childhood Illness

He will bless those who fear the Lord – small and great alike.
May the Lord cause you to flourish, both you and your children.
May you be blessed by the Lord, the Maker of heaven and earth.
Psalm 115:13-15

Nothing pulls at a parent's heartstrings like a sick child. When our son became unexplainably ill at two years of age, my husband and I were distressed to no end. What started out as any virus might, progressed to unending leg pain and difficulty walking. Night terrors (which we at first thought were seizures) and continuous low-grade fevers went on and on. Having been raised by a nurse, I grew up toughing it out through common illnesses, and so I was an unusual first-time mom who did not run to the doctor every time my son sneezed. However, this was different, and I determined to make sure the doctors knew it. Months later and after much heartache, the illness thankfully passed, and it was theorized that he simply had a virus that targeted his legs.

Having been through such an experience, I can imagine the immeasurable grief that parents of sick children endure day after day as they watch the ongoing suffering of their precious child. As a result, I have debated over whether to include anything on children in this book.

I cringe at the thought of writing anything that might discourage the weary souls, slugging it out in the trenches.

However, in researching epigenetics I discovered a wealth of information that, although it provides a strong cautionary warning, it also brings hope for parents. Remember, epigenetic changes are inherited BUT changeable.[cxcix] The research also supports the biblical principle of health that **a child's well-being is closely tied to his or her parents.**

Keep in mind, though, that because this field of science is recent (primarily since 2003), each study done reveals the need for further study in multiple directions, suggesting that the scope of and causes for epigenetic change are vast. Many, many questions remain unanswered, including, in particular, questions related to what extent epigenetic changes are reversible. Recognizing these limitations in knowledge, I will present what is currently known so that I might augment the arsenals of parents who fight for the health of their children.

Epigenetic Tendency Towards Obesity

Although it might seem odd to begin with epigenetic research focused on obesity, the studies in this area provide some big-picture realities regarding the close link between parents and the health of their children. An unusual human case study presented itself, thanks to the meticulous study and vast medical records of the Dutch going back to the 1900s. During the last winter of World War II, the Germans prevented food and fuel transports into Amsterdam, causing a brief but severe famine resulting in 20,000 deaths.[98] After the Netherlands had recovered from the famine, extensive blood samples from the surviving population were taken and preserved.

Decades later, L.H. Lumey, an epidemiologist at Columbia University, began studying the Dutch blood samples. He also gathered current blood samples from the middle-aged survivors who had been

---

[cxcix] For an explanation of epigenetics, refer to chapter 19.

born to mothers pregnant during the famine. A decade later, following the onset of epigenetic research, Lumey was able to produce a gold-mine of hard evidence that starvation greatly impacts the epigenetic landscape of fathers to be, pregnant mothers, and their unborn children.[99]

It turns out that those born to mothers pregnant at the time of the Dutch Hunger Winter grew up to be heavier and to have higher triglyceride and LDL cholesterol levels. Of greater concern, though, was that they also had higher rates of obesity, diabetes, and schizophrenia than their counterparts.

Lumey and his colleagues then began studying hundreds of thousands of death records from those who had lived through the famine, and discovered they had a ten percent increase in mortality after age 68 as compared with those not born to mothers who lived through the famine.[100] Finally, taking advantage of new technology, Lumey most recently studied methyl groups on DNA (one of three types of epigenetic markers) from the previous blood samples. The results pinpointed many specific genes and markers impacted by the famine, which explained the negative health impacts he had observed.

A 2018 rat study that focused on determining the impact to offspring of a maternal high-fat diet (HFD) found that the epigenetic changes produced by such a diet alter the rats' biologic reward system (dopamine levels) causing addictive-like behaviors and obesity, but only through the pregnant mother or the paternal lineage.[101] [102] They discovered that these particular rats had a much higher preference for food, alcohol, and drugs (cocaine) compared to the rats in the control group.

Interestingly, by the third generation, the inherited dopamine changes diverged in males and females. The males became more likely to overeat, whereas the females became more prone to drug and alcohol addictions. A definite link has now been demonstrated through multiple studies that indicate both too much or too little food produce epigenetic changes resulting in obesity and other deleterious health conditions.

Trauma Induces Epigenetic Change

The close tie between the parents' lives and their offspring's health shows itself, not only in the area of nutrition but also with stress and trauma. Following the World Trade Center attacks on September 11, 2001, Dr. Rachel Yahuda was asked to study the surviving, pregnant mothers and their babies to see whether the traumatic event had any effect on the unborn child. As the professor of psychiatry and neuroscience and the director of the Traumatic Stress Studies Division at the Mount Sinai School of Medicine, Yahuda has focused much of her life's work on understanding the impact trauma has on individuals.

Cortisol levels provide one measurable indicator of Post Traumatic Stress Disorder (PTSD) and can be monitored easily through saliva. Both the mothers and their year-old babies had multiple saliva tests done to determine if their results correlated and reflected PTSD. Indeed, the infant's cortisol levels did mirror those seen in the mothers indicating the trauma had affected the baby's epigenome while still in the womb. These results support other studies that suggest the stress response from trauma can be passed down from mother to child during pregnancy.[103]

Psychologists have long understood that traumatic experiences can produce behavioral disorders that are often passed to offspring. According to Isabelle Mansuy, a professor at ETH Zurich and the University of Zurich, *There are diseases, such as bipolar disorder, that run in families but can't be traced back to a particular gene.*[104] However, studies on epigenetics now shed light on this old conundrum.

For instance, stress has been found to alter one type of epigenetic marker, microRNAs. Mansuy's team studied numerous types of microRNAs, whose tasks include regulating the formation of proteins that influence the expression of DNA. In rat studies, they discovered that stress alters the number of many types of microRNAs found in blood, the brain, and sperm.[105] These imbalances not only affected the rat's stress response but also their metabolism, insulin, and blood-sugar levels into the third generation. Human studies reveal similar results.[106]

Epigenetic Tendency Towards Depression

After meeting at a bar while attending an international conference on neurobiology, a long-term partnership developed between Moshe Szyf, a molecular biologist and geneticist, and Michael Meaney, a neurobiologist. Together these men have now researched and published over two-dozen papers on epigenetics, including their landmark paper, *Epigenetic Programming by Maternal Behavior* in Nature Neuroscience in 2004.

Rather than looking at microRNAs, they have focused their epigenetic research on DNA methylation. Szyf says, *Methyl groups work like a placeholder in a cookbook, attaching to the DNA within each cell to select only those recipes — er, genes — necessary for that particular cell's proteins.*[107] Too much or too little DNA methylation and problems arise, as methylation suppresses genes that should be turned on (i.e. genes that suppress tumor growth) or turns on genes that need to be suppressed (i.e., genes related to handling stress).[cc]

In 2009, Szyf and Meaney published a study comparing the brains of suicide victims who had been abused as children with those who had died suddenly from something other than suicide and who had not been abused as children. *They found excess methylation of genes in the suicide brain's hippocampus, a region critical to memory acquisition and stress response.*[108] Although numerous other studies have been done on the post-mortem brains of suicide victims, only those of individuals who had been known to suffer childhood abuse consistently showed the increased epigenetic changes in methyl groups.[109] This provides yet another indicator that significant stressors in childhood increase DNA methylation and result in long-term epigenetic changes.

A Child's Necessary Buffer

[cc] DNA methylation is to be distinguished from cellular methylation, which is necessary for detoxification and other "housekeeping" processes necessary for health.

In 2017, Szyf and colleagues from Yale University published a human study comparing blood from Russian children--14 raised in orphanages and 14 who were not. Those raised in orphanages showed significantly more methylation. In particular, methyl groups that greatly influence neural communication and brain development and function were increased.[110] The results demonstrate what many previous studies with animals have revealed: The presence and amount of maternal care are highly responsible for the epigenetic regulation of genes involved in the control of the hypothalamic–pituitary–adrenal system.[111] In other words, a mother's care has a profound impact on the health and well-being of the child.

During World War II, children were often removed from their parents in an attempt to protect them from the war itself or from the Holocaust. These efforts were heroic and required great sacrifice by parents and others, and they saved the lives of many children. Unfortunately, the negative impact of parental separation on those children now appears to have been tremendous and lasting. Mental illness and many other types of health issues arose throughout the lives of the children separated from their parents during the war.[112]

Nim Tottenham, a psychology professor at Columbia University and an expert in emotional development explains why children suffer profoundly from being separated from their parents.

A parent is really in many ways an extension of the child's biology as that child is developing. That adult who's routinely been there provides this enormous stress-buffering effect on a child's brain at a time when we haven't yet developed that for ourselves. They're really one organism, in a way.[113]

I recently saw evidence of that "stress-buffering effect" as I stood waiting for my ride at an airport. I watched a nearby infant who hung in a pouch on his mother's belly with his tiny arms and legs dangling free. Unfortunately, he hung facing forwards. He could see the chaos of the world all around but not his mother's face. Someone would walk by or a car would honk, and he, with alarm in his eyes, would attempt to look for his mother's face.   She, oblivious to her son's need, continuously typed on her phone. It became quite apparent that he was looking for reassurance from his mother to learn if the tumult before him was cause for concern. He clearly did not know how to interpret the bustling world that accosted his senses.

Any person observant of children has surely seen similar scenarios. Just picture a child clinging to his parent's leg as he or she stares out, with big eyes, at the world passing by. The child constantly looks up to the parent for eye contact, reassurance, and coaching on how to handle the situation before him or her.   As Tottenham explained, this behavior is necessary because a child's brain has not yet developed and therefore relies on the parent to buffer the world. Remove or significantly limit this buffer, and the child will suffer.

A Biblical Perspective

The Bible speaks of children close to five hundred times but does not offer any definitive instruction on their health. However, if you read these passages mentioning children, you begin to see that in God's economy, children are an extension of their parents. What happens to the parents, happens to the children. For example, Proverbs 14:26 says, ***Whoever fears the LORD has a secure fortress, and for their children it will be a refuge.***

Psalm 115:13-15 speaks of the LORD blessing the parents and their children and causing them both to flourish. Numerous other passages warn that if parents rebel against God, both they and their children will suffer the consequences.[cci] Biblically speaking, the parent and child go hand in hand.

As discussed in the last chapter, Ezekiel 18 repeatedly and explicitly explains that God will not punish the children for the sins of the fathers or vice versa. When the child suffers harm because of the

---

[cci] 2 Chronicles 30:9, Deuteronomy 5:29 and 6:1-3, Jeremiah 32:18, Hosea 4:6

parent's sin, the impact on the child is not due to God specifically punishing the child for the parent's sin. Instead, harm comes because of the simple reality that the child must rely in all regards, including developmentally, on the parent. Therefore, the parents' status, good or bad, determines the health and well-being of their offspring. Epigenetics explains, biologically, one way this occurs.

For example, if Mom frets and worries continually rather than trusting God with her circumstances, the child will, by extension, not have an adequate stress-buffer. This turns up negative genetic expression through epigenetic markers. Frances Champagne, a scientist and associate professor at Columbia University, has focused her research on the impact of a mother's nurturing on a child's epigenome. She says, *The thing I've gained from the work I do is that stress is a big suppressor of maternal behavior.*[114] So, if Mom is anxious and stressed, she will not be able to mother optimally. As I will explain shortly, DNA methylation greatly increases when nurturing is minimized.

Husbands and fathers also play an equally important role in affecting their children's health. By providing stability, strength, and support to the wife and mother, he decreases her stress, empowering her to be a more nurturing mother. A man's less emotional approach to life can also provide a stable stress-buffer to children, unless he chooses to frequently walk in sinful behaviors like angry outbursts, addictions, selfishness, working too much, and so on. As the God-ordained head of the family, the man has great power to provide a secure fortress for his family.

To date, studies in epigenetics strongly indicate that bad lifestyle choices, poor diet, addictions, toxins, extreme poverty or wealth, separation from parents, childhood abuse, and multiple other stressors all increase epigenetic markers, thereby turning up the volume on negative gene expression. Although studies, obviously, do not consider the spiritual impact of sin on epigenetics, the above list provides sufficient indication that a parent's sinful patterns will impact the health of the child. If you have a sick child, I encourage you to ask the Lord to search your heart to reveal patterns of sin that might possibly be affecting your child's health. Remember, *a heart at peace gives life to the body,*[ccii] and the peace of your child greatly rests with you.

The news of a parent's effect on the epigenome of the child might be disheartening if such changes were always irreversible. After all, we are all sinners living in a fallen world. No parent is perfect. Thankfully, God, in His great mercy, placed within human biology the capability for reversing prior damage. Although scientific study does not yet understand or know the limits to the possibility for change, change does happen. Dan Hurley, author of *Grandma's Experiences Leave a Mark on Your Genes* eloquently writes,

> *Like grandmother's vintage dress, you could wear it or have it altered. The genome has long been known as the blueprint of life, but the epigenome is life's Etch A Sketch: Shake it hard enough, and you can wipe clean the family curse.*[115]

Nature Versus Nurture

Powerful evidence of nurture overriding nature is seen with surrogate mothers. Until recent years, only anecdotal evidence existed of an astonishing phenomenon in the children of surrogate mothers and egg donors--that the children, although genetically different from the mother, acquire genetic traits of the mother. In 2015 a landmark study by Dr. Carlos Simon, Ph.D. and his colleagues was published, confirming past suspicions.[116] Simon reported,

> *It turns out molecules known as microRNAs that are secreted in the mother's womb act as a communication system between the mother (or surrogate) and the growing fetus. The endometrial milk nurtures the embryos, but it is also involved in gene regulation.*[117]

[ccii] Proverbs 14:30

The incredible fact that a non-genetic mother can actually alter the expression of a child's DNA to mimic her own brings to the forefront the old debate over which has a stronger influence, nature or nurture? Psychologist David S. Moore, Ph.D. addresses this question in, The Developing Genome;

> *For the longest time, the nature-nurture debate has been cast as a kind of contest between genes and experiences. The thought was that we might have some characteristics that are caused primarily by genetic factors and other characteristics that are caused primarily by experiential factors.*
>
> *What epigenetics is making clear is that's a faulty way to think about the situation, because it's not true that genes do things independently of their contexts.* ***Instead, genes do what they do because of the contexts that they're in. Nature and nurture are always working together to produce all of our traits.***[118]

The Power of Nurturing on Epigenetics

In epigenetics, timing is everything. Although the two primary periods for the formation of the epigenome are conception and pregnancy, scientific studies now reveal that significant changes during early childhood also have a profound impact.[119] It is during childhood that a mother's tender affection toward her child can impart lasting health.

Often in science, what initially appears to be the cause for a particular outcome proves false upon further study. Such was the case in a rat study by Michael Meaney in which baby rats were handled by humans, causing the pups to grow up to be healthier than their non-handled counterparts. In actuality, human handling simply caused the mother rats to incessantly lick their pups and nurse them in a way that allowed for closer contact.

Upon further study, Meaney determined that this significant increase in the mothers' nurturing behaviors produced positive epigenetic changes in the rat pups, who also later became more nurturing mothers to their offspring.[120] The conclusions were obvious. Nurturing had a direct impact on DNA methylation. The licking and close nursing worked like a dimmer switch, and in this case, turned down the expression of stress hormone production into adulthood and eventually into the third generation.[121]

From studying the brains of well-nurtured pups, they discovered almost no DNA methylation in the areas that deal with stress. In contrast, they found highly methylated brains in their unnurtured counterparts. With still further study, they determined that cross-fostering pups who had higher methylation in the first week of life, with more nurturing mothers reversed their methylation. The corresponding positive epigenetic changes also persisted into adulthood.

The abstract concludes with the statement; *Thus we show that an epigenomic state of a gene can be established through behavioral programming, and it is potentially reversible.*[122] The impact of this knowledge is huge! Mothers, the amount that you nurture your children directly and powerfully improves your children's epigenome and, therefore, their health. If there has been prior damage or bad genetics, your maternal affection could potentially reverse or dial-down the volume of that genetic expression.

Frances Champagne, who once worked in Meaney's lab, discovered that the brains of rat pups raised by less nurturing mothers have greater DNA methylation on estrogen receptors. As a result, the female offspring grew up to be less nurturing mothers as well.[123]

If you were raised by a not-so-nurturing or absent mother, then you may struggle with demonstrating affection and tender care for your own children. Although you came by this tendency through no fault of your own, continuing to walk according to the sinful inheritance that was passed down to you is your choice alone. I say, sinful, because the numerous references in the Bible to a mother's comfort, compassion, and care, as well as the instruction to be such a mother, indicate that God intends moms to nurture and affectionately love their children.[cciii]

If affection and tender care for your children does not come naturally, do not lose heart. Like with any sin, repentance is at hand. I encourage you to do three things: First, apply the teaching (at the end of the last chapter) on not walking according to the sins of the fathers but according to the new life the Spirit provides IN Christ. You are not a slave to the past.

Second, it might be helpful to write on note cards the verses on mothering that I put in the footnote below so that you can place them in key places. Doing so makes it easier to meditate on those Scriptures and to make them a part of your prayers as you go about your day and interact with your children.

You might even take some time to make a list of specific opportunities that frequently arise or ones you can intentionally create with your children in order to increase your affection and tender care. For example, when giving a baby his bottle, make time to hold the child close and look in his eyes while talking or singing to him instead of placing him on his own to eat while you do something else. Touch and eye contact are so important! When children begin attending school, getting them groomed and out the door can be a frantic endeavor. However, after they return home or at bedtime, a nurturing mother can find many opportunities to incorporate affection--brushing a girl's hair, snuggling while reading a book, caressing a boy's head as he lays in bed before going to sleep, etc.

Tender affection becomes more difficult as a child ages, but the need and importance still continue, requiring thoughtful strategy at

---

[cciii] Isaiah 66:13 *As a mother comforts her child, so will I comfort you.*
Isaiah 49:15 *Can a mother forget the baby at her breast and have no compassion on the child she has borne? Though she may forget, I will not forget you!*
1 Thessalonians 2:7 *...Just as a nursing mother cares for her children...*
Titus 2:4 *Then they can train the younger women to love their husbands and love their children...*

times. For example, when my son entered the teenage years, strife between us increased and hugs became more awkward. After thinking about our routine, I came up with an idea that worked. I found that he really liked it if I would position myself so that I could rub his shoulders or head while we daily read the Bible as a family. Every family's routine, as well as every child's preferences, will be different, but thinking through those specifics will reveal opportunities to make nurturing affection a regular part of your mothering.

Third, if you currently are a mother with a schedule that robs you of time and energy so that you are too stressed and exhausted to be nurturing to your children, I urge you to seriously pray about what God would have you do to change that situation. Your physical presence and expressed love are powerful forces in your children's ability to thrive.

Sarah's Story

I would like to end the chapter by sharing a story that illustrates the real-life impact of a mother's love and the Lord's mercy on a child with a severe genetic condition. Sarah, a close friend and fellow sister in Christ, has shared with me the actual medical records of her son so that I might more accurately portray their story.

Three years ago, Sarah shared with me the news of her second pregnancy. What should have been a joyous report was not. Her husband, an addict, had begun using again, and they were living with their baby girl in Sarah's mother's home. Thankfully, before long her husband entered rehab, but the future loomed like an approaching storm. To make matters significantly worse, problems with the pregnancy indicated from the beginning that something was very wrong. Unexplained things like extreme water retention and an alarming increase in the size of her baby's brain ventricles set the stage for the unique and consuming needs that this baby would bring into their lives. Following the birth of Landon on June 11, 2016, concerned doctors placed him on oxygen in the NICU ward for the first week of his life.

Landon, now two-and-a-half years old, has the sole distinction of being the only person in recorded history to have his unique genetic condition. A mere handful of children have similar chromosomal disorders, but none match his condition exactly. His unbalanced, genetic translocation falls between chromosomes 5 and 7. The complete genetic microarray reveals 140 affected genes, many of which are associated with disease, structural abnormalities, heart and brain problems, and the list goes on and on. As a result of Landon's uniqueness, the vast team of doctors who have diligently worked to provide him with the highest possible level of care, have often found themselves shooting in the dark to fix the problems that, at first, arose with alarming regularity.

Sarah seemed to spend more time at Children's National Hospital fighting for her son's life than at home. Because Landon could not swallow or breathe properly, he frequently aspirated milk and later food, causing frequent bouts of pneumonia. First, a feeding tube was placed through his nose, but when tiny hands managed to repeatedly pull it out, a G-tube was inserted directly into his stomach. Because food continued to reflux and then be aspirated, the doctor resorted to placing a GJ-tube directly into his small intestine in an attempt to bypass the stomach altogether.

With a weak immune system and breathing difficulties that required constant oxygen, every germ proved a formidable threat, requiring another lengthy hospital stay. Among his many alarming symptoms was screaming. For no apparent reason, Landon would frequently arch his back and scream as though in torturous pain. Every test imaginable was performed and then repeated, each one showing more areas of concern but offering no direction or explanation for the blood-curdling cries. Doctors encouraged Sarah to avoid moving or holding her son because touch often seemed to upset him. Yet, between the episodes of screaming and sickness, the little boy with a thick mop of sandy, brown hair smiled frequently and stole the hearts of all those around him.

I will never forget receiving a call from Sarah, just days before Christmas. Hospice had been called in, and Landon's first Christmas would likely be his last. This devoted mother found herself torn between a longing for her precious son to live and a desire for his suffering to cease. On receipt of that phone call, I just cried out to the Lord to heal him. Miraculously, Landon made it through that Christmas.

Life for Landon involved every type of therapy imaginable, and yet doctors regularly reminded Sarah that he would probably never talk or walk or do any of the things most parents take for granted with their children. Managing her days proved challenging with one child barely hanging on to life while the other, an almost three-year-old daughter, exuded life from every fiber of her being. When Landon was around a year old and after many months of therapies bringing no noticeable improvements, a new neurologist recommended a significant change in their approach.

Instead of Sarah focusing on forcing her little boy to do specific exercises, the doctor instructed her to just start talking to him all of the time and making sure he accompanied her wherever she went around the house. "Start holding him more" was the new instruction. Because he was usually hooked up to oxygen and monitors, moving him was a chore, and so Sarah had often kept him in one place.

After five or six months of the new approach, noticeable improvements began. Landon started getting sick less and gradually needed less oxygen until none was needed. He could eat through his mouth instead of the GJ-tube. The little man began holding his head up and can now even sit up by himself.

To the tremendous surprise of the doctors and the great joy of Sarah, he recently said his first word, "Mama." When I telephoned Sarah to question her about some of her story for this chapter, I could hear the precious sound of Landon in the background, babbling away like any child learning to talk, and saying "Mama" repeatedly with great clarity. He apparently also likes to add, "My Mama" and "up Mama" to his conversation. Oh, how remarkable these changes truly are!

It was finally discovered that the cause of his screaming as an infant was likely due to constant ear infections. Since he no longer required a Bi-pap machine (a ventilator) at night, he could have surgery done to remove his adenoids and put in ear tubes, thereby ending the infections.

The doctor suspected hearing loss, and so a standard hearing assessment was made, which revealed more cause for concern. While Landon was under sedation for the insertion of ear tubes, the most accurate hearing test available revealed moderate to severe sensorineural and conductive hearing loss.[cciv] He was measured for a Baja headband (a headset hearing aid) that he would wear until his teenage years, when he could then switch to hearing aids for the rest of his life. Sarah called me heartbroken with the news. Of all the problems her son had endured, the hearing loss troubled her the most. "Why would God let such a thing happen," she asked? For two years, while every test known to man was done on her son, the doctors missed something so simple and fixable as ear infections, which left untreated, caused irreversible conductive damage. (The sensorineural hearing loss was brain related and likely stemmed from some other aspect of his condition.)

I grieved with her at the news but began to intercede daily on her behalf. "Lord, please have mercy on Sarah and Landon. I don't know why you allowed this but please glorify yourself by healing his hearing completely." Before the expensive hearing contraption could arrive but after trying a loaner set, Landon had the regular hearing test repeated, and the results were shocking. The new test showed him to be barely

---

[cciv] Sensorineural hearing loss results from damage to the inner ear or to the nerve pathways that lead from the inner ear to the brain. Conductive hearing loss occurs when something is blocking sound waves from reaching the inner ear, through the outer and middle ear.

within the normal range of hearing. Elated, Sarah called me with the news. I told her what I had been praying and asked her to join me in praying for the complete healing of his hearing.

Shortly thereafter, Landon had surgery done to remove his adenoids, and so the sedation hearing test was repeated. This time, a mystified doctor announced that Landon's significant hearing loss had completely disappeared. He now had perfect hearing! He could even hear the gentle plunk of a water drop. When Sarah asked the doctor how this could happen, he confessed to having no idea. With great joy, she declared that she knew. "God did it!" she exclaimed. As Jesus said in reference to the healing of a blind man, ***This happened so that the works of God might be displayed in him.***[ccv]

Current diagnostic tests still indicate problems of all kinds, including serious concerns with Landon's brain. He has both white matter and brainstem loss, which should be affecting his breathing, swallowing, balance, speech, and so on. Yet, doctors are amazed at how the little guy can do all that he does, and every day continues to bring new developmental progress. With conviction, Landon's pediatrician simply stated, "It's you, Sarah." It appears that, by God's grace, the simple acts of a mother's nurturing love have dialed down the genetic expression of a host of symptoms that Landon's condition causes. The future, once bleak, now looks promising.

Conclusion

The new science of epigenetics is beginning to reveal that parents have a tremendous influence on the health of their children before they are ever conceived, in pregnancy, in childhood, into adulthood, and into subsequent generations. This supports the biblical principle that **a child's well-being is closely tied to his or her parents.** I am certainly not suggesting that childhood illness is always related to the close tie between parent and child or that a parent has the power to make a sick

---

[ccv] John 9:3

child well. As with any means that might bring healing, ultimately, God is the Great Physician who can make something (or someone) effective or ineffective.

In the Bible, outright healing of children always came about through the parent as the child's advocate.[ccvi] You too can be your child's advocate to the Great Physician who loves His children. To be an effective intercessor for your children, though, you must be at peace with God, walking in the righteousness of Christ. Let nothing interfere with this. Often the needs of chronically ill children lead a parent to neglect these areas. Although the gracious Father remembers our human frailties and understands our struggles, only He has the power to heal. Therefore, the needy parent should remember the importance of maintaining that relationship. The words found in Deuteronomy 30:19-20 speak strongly of the impact that following the LORD has on the whole family.

> *This day I call the heavens and the earth as witnesses against you that I have set before you life and death, blessings and curses. Now choose life, so that you and your children may live and that you may love the Lord your God, listen to his voice, and hold fast to him. For the Lord is your life.*

As a parent seeks the Lord, He blesses both parent and child. God can then work according to His will to breathe life into your child's body, through His Spirit, whether it be through medical intervention, epigenetic change, or an outright miracle.[ccvii] May God bless you and your children!

[ccvi] Matthew 15:21-28, Matthew 9:18-23, 1 Kings 17:17-23,
[ccvii] Romans 8:6

Biblical Principle: *A child's well-being is closely tied to his or her parents.*

Call to Action: *Ask the Lord to search your heart to see if there are any patterns of sin that require repentance, whose effects might be spilling over into your children's lives.*[ccviii]

Find ways, if needed, to increase the level of maternal care for your children. No one can take a mother's place.

Personally intercede diligently for your children, confident that God listens to parents.

[ccviii] Hosea 4:6

CHAPTER 21

Conclusion

Do not be wise in your own eyes; fear the LORD and shun evil.
This will bring health to your body and nourishment to your
bones. Proverbs 3:7-8

The end was in sight. After two years of writing, my final sprint began to complete the task of writing this book. Then it happened; I got sick. The excruciating pain in my left flank alerted me to the frightfully slow journey of a kidney stone as it passed. Who knew that something so small could, not only cause pain on par with delivering a baby but also produce all-consuming nausea. Three and a half weeks later it finally passed, but the misery persisted. A kidney infection had set in, and so I began a round of antibiotics. Since I had not taken antibiotics in ten years, they worked quickly, but then the pain, nausea, and weakness started up again. The doctor seemed mystified.

Seek to Know God

In knowing the first two principles of health-- **God desires that we diligently seek His direction regarding our health** and **God's Word contains knowledge of the path of life (health)**, I set aside a day for prayer and fasting. Although doctors and medicine can be a blessing at times, they so often fall short of bringing relief, hope, and healing. Furthermore, the stories of kings Asa and Hezekiah reveal God's desire that mankind might earnestly seek Him for every need, especially when it comes to illness. We cannot know how often God has blocked the way to wellness when individuals will not humble themselves and seek Him instead of physicians, but we know from Asa's story that God does just that.[ccix]

In our information age, we generally respond to symptoms by scouring the internet for knowledge on our condition. The prophet Hosea spoke of God's people perishing because they lacked knowledge, but it was not earthly knowledge they lacked. They needed the knowledge of God and His ways. The same is true today. Christians often spend minimal to no time reading and studying the Bible, and yet we are told that healing knowledge comes through the Word of God. *He sent out his word and healed them; he rescued them from the grave.*[ccx]

The sick are wise when they humble themselves and seek, with great earnestness, to know the Creator and Sustainer of life through His Word. Perhaps like me, you could benefit from a day of prayer and fasting, or perhaps what is needed is a general change to spending more time in God's presence on a daily basis. Regardless, the simple words of Psalm 119:144 make a fitting prayer. It says, *Your statutes are forever right; give me understanding that I may live.*

I am a list person who loves the sense of accomplishment that comes when I can cross through completed tasks. However, the biblical path of life does not work that way. Just as Christianity is a relationship with the Savior, so also the path of life flows out of that relationship. Psalm 16:11 says, *You have made known to me the path of life. You will fill me with joy in your presence.* In knowing God, we discover the path of life. King Solomon speaks at length in Proverbs 3-6 of the path of life being a continuous journey with God's

[ccix] 2 Chronicles 16:12-13
[ccx] Psalm 107:20

truth as the roadmap. When one walks this path, the positive impact on health is evident.

> *My son, do not forget my teaching, but keep my commands in your heart, for they will prolong your life many years and bring you peace and prosperity... Trust in the LORD with all your heart and lean not on your own understanding; in all your ways submit to him, and he will make your paths straight. Do not be wise in your own eyes; fear the LORD and shun evil. This will bring health to your body and nourishment to your bones.*

> *My son, do not despise the LORD's discipline, and do not resent his rebuke, because the LORD disciplines those he loves, as a father the son he delights in. Do not let them* (wisdom) *out of your sight, keep them within your heart; for they are life to those who find them and health to a man's whole body. Above all else, guard your heart, for it is the wellspring of life.* (Proverbs 3:1-2, 5-8, 11-12, 4:21-23)

The Common Versus Biblical View of Health

As a result of all my studies, my response to illness noticeably differs from the average person. The following chart depicts how Christians typically view health.

God

the spirit realm, of
which God is control

The Heart

spirit & soul

The Physical

diet, exercise, genetics, germs, etc.

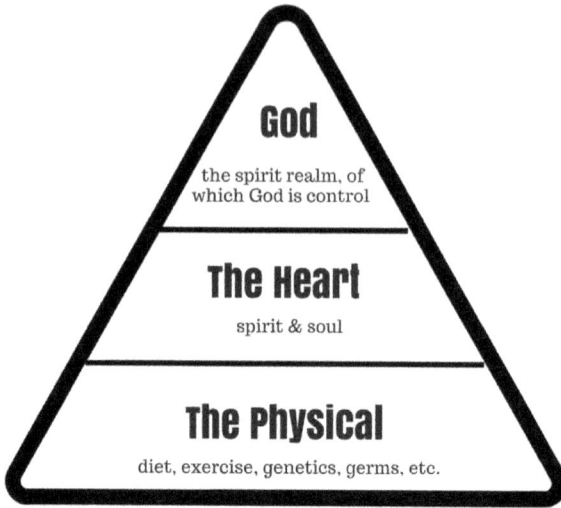

Common Perspective of Health

chart created by Marci Julin--HeartandMindMinistries.com

It is assumed that everything in the physical realm has the greatest impact. With this as the foundation for health, the seemingly logical reasoning is that if something affects you in the physical realm, the solution must also be found through physical means. So, medical intervention, diet, exercise, etc. become the focus.

However, the biblical perspective of health reverses what people commonly assume. God or the spirit realm has the greatest impact, with the heart following in importance. All the physical components, whether diet, exercise, germs, or genetics, influence health to the degree that God and the heart allow.

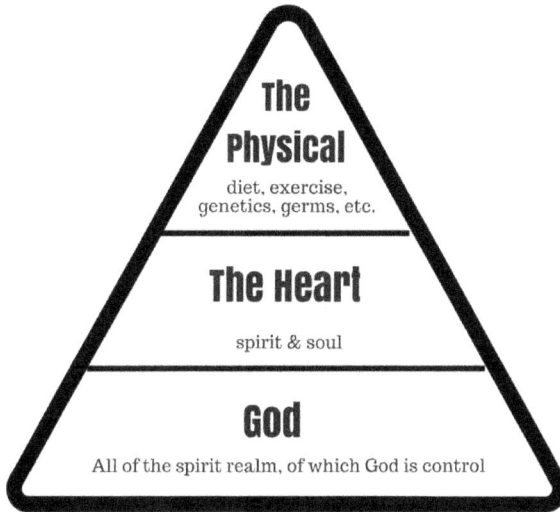

The
Physical
diet, exercise,
genetics, germs, etc.

The Heart

spirit & soul

God

All of the spirit realm, of which God is control

A Biblical Perspective of Health

chart created by Marci Julin--HeartandMindMinistries.com

As Paul said, *For physical training is of some value, but godliness has value for all things.*[ccxi] Because God has the power to bless or block the way to health, and the heart gives or hinders life, everything in the physical realm can be effective or ineffective depending on factors outside of that realm. Understanding and applying that knowledge brings a complete paradigm shift in how one approaches illness.

The biblical perspective of health reveals a direct connection between the physical and the spiritual. We see this connection most clearly when peace with God is missing. As a result, the Father may use illness as a tool of discipline for sin. The other reality depicted biblically is that when we walk according to the flesh rather than the Spirit, we hinder our source of life, the Holy Spirit. Last, we also discover the spiritual effecting the physical upon reading of the

---

[ccxi] 1 Timothy 4:8

numerous ill people in the Bible whose symptoms and illnesses were linked directly to the spirit realm.

All of the following are cases attributed to spirits: Job had boils from head to toe. Children had seizures (Matthew 17:15-18). A man was mute (Matthew 9:32-33) and a woman was crippled for 18 years (Luke 13:10-16). Acts 5:16 speaks of the *sick and those tormented by evil spirits* being *healed,* and 19:12 also says that *their illnesses were cured and the evil spirits left them.* Therefore, the Bible clearly contradicts the assumption that all physical symptoms are from physical causes. Furthermore, Ephesians 6:11-12 reminds us that the seemingly physical struggle we face is actually a spiritual one.

> *Put on the full armor of God, so that you can take your stand against the devil's schemes·* *For our struggle is not against flesh and blood, but against the rulers, against the authorities, against the powers of this dark world and against the spiritual forces of evil in the heavenly realms.*

Therefore, if healing has not come, I urge you to begin by determining why the spiritual is negatively influencing the physical. Is peace lacking with God, self, or others?

The Heart and the Flesh

As I agonized over my ongoing kidney symptoms, I again read the chapters focused on the principles that **out of the heart (soul and spirit) flows life** and **the path of life is peace.** These chapters reminded me of an important truth: Regardless of the cause or reason for continued illness, the emotional and spiritual state of the heart will either breathe life into every cell of the body or hinder the healing process. Therefore, one very important question begs an answer--Is my heart at peace with God, myself, and others?

In sickness or in pain, the sin-nature can easily take control as one's focus naturally centers around the needs of the body. Self-preservation at any cost often becomes the knee-jerk reaction to everything. Satan would have us walk in this realm of the flesh, and the self-absorption sickness demands makes us vulnerable to those fleshly desires of the soul. A vicious and self-perpetuating cycle of giving in to the sin nature can easily rob us of our source of life.

According to Scripture, **to walk according to the flesh brings death but to walk according to the Spirit brings life and peace.** By tracing the thread of the flesh throughout the Bible in chapter 12, we saw that this truth about the flesh is literal. The flesh brings sin and death, but the Spirit brings life and peace. Romans 8:13 summarizes the matter by saying, ***For if you live according to the flesh you will die, but if by the Spirit you put to death the deeds of the body, you will live.*** Do we want life and peace? Then, we must allow the Holy Spirit to govern our hearts, not the flesh.[ccxii]

When I cannot seem to break out of the cycle of walking according to the flesh, I find it very helpful to fast.[ccxiii] By purposefully denying the flesh, I silence the clamor of fleshly demands that I might better hear the Spirit's gentle voice. He then reveals sin so that I might repent and restore peace with God, myself, and others. Even if God's discipline for sin is not the cause of the illness, turning the focus from the misery of the flesh to the Spirit who gives life is exceedingly valuable. God will not despise a broken and contrite heart.[ccxiv]

Repentance and Healing

My kidney pain continued into the fifth week, so I earnestly sought to listen to the conviction of the Holy Spirit and to pray that God might reveal if His discipline was at the root of my symptoms. The check engine light was on, and I needed to know why. Just as there can be many reasons that a car's warning light might come on, so also there can be many reasons for illness in God's children. However,

---

[ccxii] Romans 8:6, *The mind governed by the flesh is death, but the mind governed by the Spirit is life and peace.*
[ccxiii] For more information on fasting, see Appendix H.
[ccxiv] Psalm 51:7

since the vast majority of passages on illness in the Bible speak of **illness as a tool of discipline used by the loving Heavenly Father to sanctify His children**, it is wise to respond to the warning light of physical suffering by earnestly requesting that the Lord reveal any sin at the root of the disease.

If conviction comes, the promise that **true repentance leads to healing from illness** provides great hope. **Jesus' suffering at the cross conquered the curse of the flesh (death) making provision through sanctification so that we can be healed.** The work has been done. Provision has been made.

God spoke powerfully on repentance bringing healing through Ezekiel in 18:30-32

> *Repent! Turn away from all your offenses; then sin will not be your downfall. Rid yourselves of all the offenses you have committed, and get a new heart and a new spirit. Why will you die, people of Israel? For I take no pleasure in the death of anyone, declares the Sovereign Lord. Repent and live!*

Because God does not treat us as our sins deserve, He often allows much time to pass before disciplining for sin. I fear that His patience, intended to give us an opportunity to repent of our own accord, instead causes us to fail to make the connection between our sin and the Lord's discipline.

The Reason Many Are Not Healed

Many believers wrestle with understanding why a loving and good God allows so many of His children to suffer endlessly with pain and illness. I have heard and read many explanations of this, of which I imagine you are also familiar. Some say it is because, in our weakness, God is strong and therefore glorified. I would not argue with this truth as stated by Paul in 2 Corinthians 4 and 12. However, I do question a couple of assumptions regarding that teaching.

The only evidence given for this assumption originates with another assumption, which is that the "thorn in the flesh" that Paul three times asked for God to remove was a medical problem.[ccxv] However, Paul used the term "flesh" repeatedly in his writings to refer to the sin nature. Therefore, concluding that his "thorn in the flesh" was a physical malady runs counter to his primary use of the word.

Furthermore, when you look at the context of the passage, which includes numerous chapters, one sees that Paul felt the need to defend himself against the aggressive character assassination that some individuals were conducting to discredit his work for the Gospel. It is in that context where Paul calls the thorn in the flesh *a messenger of Satan to harass me, to keep me from becoming conceited.*[ccxvi] Surely the defamation of his character raised a mighty battle in his flesh against these individuals who were truly "messengers of Satan," and that their attacks did much to keep the noble apostle humble. Therefore, I see no reason to conclude that Paul's thorn was an illness.

Another assumption people make is that because God is glorified in our weakness, His will might be for someone to be sick until they die.[ccxvii] Based on the passages on repentance leading to healing, as well as several other passages, I do greatly question that fatalistic assumption.

To the contrary, John wishes that his readers would *enjoy good health...even as your soul is getting along well,*[ccxviii] which reminds us of the role of the heart as the wellspring of life and the need for peace in the heart. Additionally, Psalm 41:3 says that God will *sustain them on their sickbed AND RESTORE them from their bed of illness.* Psalm 103:3 says, *He forgives all my sins and heals all my diseases.*

[ccxv] 2 Corinthians 11:29

[ccxvi] 2 Corinthians 12:7 ESV

[ccxvii] Psalm 90:10 says, *Our days may come to seventy years, or eighty, if our strength endures; yet the best of them are but trouble and sorrow, for they quickly pass, and we fly away.* As I taught earlier in the book, old age does typically bring illnesses that bring death, i.e., David & Elijah.

[ccxviii] 3 John 1:2

Isaiah 53:5 and 1 Peter 2:24 say, *by his wounds you are healed.* How can all these passages and others be reconciled with the teaching that God's will is that someone should be sick until they die in order to bring Himself glory? *For I take <u>no pleasure</u> in the death of anyone, declares the Sovereign Lord. Repent and live!*[ccxix]

Some argue that illness makes us more like Christ, and therefore, He allows His children to be sick to accomplish this purpose. I wholeheartedly agree that illness sanctifies us, but not in the sense that God desires sickness for His children any more than good parents desire to spank their children continuously. Spanking may serve a good purpose but is not desirable for its own sake. Discipline has a good but hopefully temporary purpose--to bring an end to wrong behavior, thinking, or attitudes. Once the pain has served its purpose for restoration, it can and should end. A conclusion that God wants to make His children sick infers that He is even less kind than parents who have a sin nature. Jesus illustrated the absurdity of such thinking in Matthew 7:9-11,

> *"Which of you, if your son asks for bread, will give him a stone" Or if he asks for a fish, will give him a snake? If you, then, though you are evil, know how to give good gifts to your children, how much more will your Father in heaven give good gifts to those who ask him!*

God may bring much good out of illness, but the illness itself is not good. He is a loving Father, not one who delights in giving painful "gifts." Furthermore, sickness is always connected to sin because of the curse and therefore is not a "gift" from the Father.

I have also heard people say that sickness is one of the many types of suffering that Paul warns will come and that we should count ourselves blessed to suffer. It might surprise you to read the multiple lists of sufferings found in the New Testament and to realize that illness

---

[ccxix] Ezekiel 18:32

is not once included.[ccxx]   Instead, Peter contrasted suffering for following Christ with suffering for bad behavior.[ccxxi] The context of these chapters, just as in the other lists, is the persecution of the church. The apostles taught that just as Christ endured persecution, so too would His followers. THAT suffering is just and to be expected. Illness is not even hinted at in those discourses.

Why, then, do so many Christians continue to be sick year after year after year, asking for healing that never comes? Some say that a lack of faith keeps healing at bay; so, they attempt to muster up the necessary measure. Still, complete healing proves elusive. They then either grow discouraged and resentful towards God, or they reconcile God's actions by determining that their illness is a badge of honor showing that they were counted worthy to suffer.

Perhaps, however, God's children frequently forfeit the blessing of healing on account of two things. First, they neglect the heart's need for peace. Second, God often uses illness to draw our attention to sin, and when He does, He will not bring healing without true repentance. Like with King Asa, God may specifically block the effectiveness of medical intervention and prevent healing. The prophet Jeremiah speaks of all these matters when he says,

> *But my people do not know the requirements of the LORD...Since they have rejected the word of the LORD, what kind of wisdom do they have?*
>
> *For they have healed the wound of my people slightly, saying "Peace, peace," when there is no peace.* (KJV) *Are they ashamed of their detestable conduct? No, they have no shame at all; they do not even know how to blush. So they will fall among the fallen; they will be brought down when they are punished, says the LORD. For the LORD our God has doomed us to perish and given us poisoned water to drink, because we have sinned*

[ccxx] 2 Corinthians 1:3-11, 11:23-29, Hebrews 10:32-39, 2 Peter 3:8-18
[ccxxi] 1 Peter 2-3

against him. We hoped for peace but no good has come, for a time of healing but there is only terror.

Is there no balm in Gilead? Is there no physician there? Why then is there no healing for the wound of my people?... Therefore this is what the LORD Almighty says: "See, I will refine and test them, for what else can I do because of the sin of my people?
(Jeremiah 8:7, 9,11-12, 15, 22 & 9:7 NIV)

During the course of writing this book, I taught some of the material at a women's Bible study.[ccxxii] After teaching the biblical principle that with true repentance comes healing and that according to Scripture God often blocks the way to healing until repentance occurs, a woman enthusiastically interrupted to share a testimony. Everyone in the group knew that Musette had been through a battle with breast cancer; however, no one knew of what had transpired during the course of her treatment.

With excitement in her voice, Musette told the group how God opened her heart during her illness. Although she said she was not depressed, she could not stop crying. Day after day, she lay on her couch remembering the sins of her life, all the way back to third grade.

For the first time, she felt true sorrow for both the big and small sins of her past. Her tears became a kind of cleansing as she confessed them to God and to others. She said she did not understand what was happening at the time, but after hearing my teaching, she realized that God had opened her eyes and led her to repentance. Because she responded, she believed He did not hinder her healing. By the time she shared her testimony, she had been cancer-free for several years.

As stated in four places where Isaiah's words are repeated fully or in part,[ccxxiii] IF God's people repent and turn from their sin, THEN they will be healed! The Hebrew word "healed" used by Isaiah means *to mend, i.e. to cure: cause to heal, physician, repair--thoroughly, make*

[ccxxii] The links to the 8 audio lessons from the *Life to the Body* series are available on my website at https://www.heartandmindministries.com/blank
[ccxxiii] Isaiah 6:9-10, Matthew 13:14, Mark 14:3, and Acts 28:26

whole.[124] Through this definition of healing, we also see the idea that healing is to be thorough--for the whole being. Healing of the whole person comes when the heart is made right through the accomplishment of Jesus at the cross and appropriated through repentance and faith.

Ask the Elders for Anointing

After a time of fasting and seeking the Lord regarding my continued kidney symptoms, I came to peace with the Spirit's reassurance that my symptoms were not the result of my heavenly Father's discipline for sin. After all, **not every illness is the result of personal sin or the absence of peace.** Instead, the Holy Spirit reminded me that I had yet to follow the admonition in James 5 that if anyone is sick, he should ask the elders for prayer and anointing so that he might be healed. This step might also include a confession of sin but not always. In response to the Spirit's prompting in this matter, I reached out to the elders of my church to ask for them to meet with me for this purpose. What a blessing my obedience to that biblical instruction proved to be.

Faith Required

The examples of healing in the Bible all indicate that the individual must have faith to be healed. Jesus praised the Canaanite woman for her great faith and in response, healed her daughter.[ccxxiv] When a man whose son was demon-possessed asked if Jesus could heal him, the response was, *"'If you can'?" said Jesus. "Everything is possible for one who believes." Immediately the boy's father exclaimed, "I do believe; help me overcome my unbelief!"*[ccxxv] Many times Jesus followed his healings with the statement, *your faith has healed you.*[ccxxvi] So, faith or trust that God can heal is required, but

---

[ccxxiv] Matthew 15:22-28
[ccxxv] Mark 9:22-24
[ccxxvi] Matthew 9:22, Mark 10:52, Luke 8:48 & 18:42

many put the cart before the horse. God brings healing according to His Word, which says, when needed, repentance comes first.

Hezekiah's Example

Earlier in this book, I spoke at length about my biblical hero, King Hezekiah. From the age of nine until he gained the throne at twenty-five, Hezekiah witnessed his father, Ahaz, despising the ways of the LORD and leading God's people increasingly more into idolatry. Although Hezekiah's grandfather Jotham had *walked steadfastly before the LORD his God*,[ccxxvii] Jotham failed to lead his people in doing the same. Therefore, the temple had long been abandoned, and even its treasures were given away by King Ahaz to Tiglath-Pileser king of Assyria.[ccxxviii]

Somehow, despite pervasive evil surrounding his upbringing, Hezekiah had a heart for God unlike any other. In the first month of his reign, he set about reinstating temple worship. Under the king's authority, the temple and its furnishings, as well as the priests and Levites were cleansed and consecrated according to the law of Moses so that they might once again fulfill their purpose.

All the required cleansings of the temple took place during the first month of the year, which happened to be the appointed time for celebrating the Passover. That sacred festival to the LORD had not been observed on a large scale for a very long time, and so it was decided that they would not wait for another year but instead celebrate the festival in the second month. Hezekiah dispatched messengers throughout the land, even unto all Israel, which was not under his jurisdiction.

Many in Judah and some in Israel journeyed to the holy city to celebrate the Passover. However, some of the people failed to follow God's commands to first consecrate themselves, and so they became ill.

[ccxxvii] 2 Chronicles 27:6
[ccxxviii] The details of this story are found in 2 Kings 16 and 2 Chronicles 29-30.

But Hezekiah prayed for them, saying, "May the LORD, who is good, pardon everyone who sets their heart on seeking God—the LORD, the God of their ancestors—even if they are not clean according to the rules of the sanctuary." And the LORD heard Hezekiah and healed the people. (2 Chronicles 30:18-20)

Countless other times in the Old Testament, God showed no mercy when His people failed to follow the letter of the law in worshipping Him. He typically did not allow leeway, and here again, we initially see that same demand for perfection under the law. So, on what basis did Hezekiah intercede on behalf of the people? The basis for his request for mercy was a heart that truly sought after God, and on that basis, God heard and healed.

I am frequently contacted by people who have heard my teaching on the biblical principles of health. With great joy, I listen to these individuals describe to me their new realization that their hearts have not been at peace in some area, and how they have chosen to turn their focus from pursuing medical knowledge and answers to their health problems to instead seeking after God. Such changes do not occur overnight. Many questions, blunders, and struggles along the way are inevitable. The fear of missing something or not doing things just right can consume the thoughts of those who want to be right with the Lord.

Because of that, I find Hezekiah's prayer and the LORD's answer to be greatly reassuring. Those people may have blundered in celebrating the Passover, but the king knew the heart of God--that His people would seek Him with all their hearts. Is that your desire? If so, keep on! Do not stop! Your heavenly Father is greatly pleased. He will hear and answer your prayer for healing. *He who promised is faithful.*[ccxxix] Go in peace.

[ccxxix] Hebrews 10:23

Appendix

Appendix A

Biblical Principles of Health

- God's Word contains knowledge of the path of life (health). (ch.1)

- God desires that we diligently seek His direction regarding our health. (ch.2)

- Out of the heart (soul and spirit) flows life. (ch.4 & 5)

- The path of life is peace. (ch.6)

- I can be transformed by the renewing of my mind by truth. (ch.7)

- Since the time of Christ, sanctification and healing have gone together. (ch.8)

- Resting in God's love brings joy and health. (ch.9)

- Illness is often a tool of discipline used by a loving heavenly Father to sanctify His children. (ch.10)

- True repentance leads to healing from illness due to sin. (ch.11)

- Jesus' suffering at the cross conquered the curse of the flesh (death) making provision through sanctification so that we can be healed. (ch.12)

- To walk according to the flesh brings death, but to walk according to the Spirit brings life and peace. (ch.13)

- Not every illness is the result of personal sin or the absence of peace. (ch.14)

- Peace with myself comes from believing God's truth about me and brings health to my whole body. (ch.15)

- God's love filling your heart must motivate you towards peace with others, bringing health and healing to your whole person. (ch.16)

- Satan uses deception to ensnare Christians through demonically based health practices. (ch.17)

- All food is good and meant by God to be a satisfying blessing. (ch.18)

- The inheritance of the fathers need not determine the health of someone who is IN Christ. (ch.19)

- A child's well-being is closely tied to his or her parents. (ch.20)

Correcting False Views of God

God loves me personally.

- Psalm 31:7, *I will be glad and rejoice in your love...*

- Psalm 36:5 & 7, *Your love, O LORD, reaches to the heavens, your faithfulness to the skies. How priceless is your unfailing love!*

- Psalm 63:3, *Because your love is better than life, my lips will glorify you.*

- Psalm 66:20, *Praise be to God, who has not rejected my prayer or withheld his love from me!*

- 1 John 3:1, *See what great love the Father has lavished on us, that we should be called the children of God! And that is what we are!*

God's love is NOT based on my performance.

- Psalm 103:13-15 & 17, *...the LORD has compassion on those who fear him, for he knows how we are formed, he remembers that we are dust. As for man, his days are like grass...But from everlasting, the LORD's love is with those who fear him.*

- Romans 5:8, *But God demonstrates his own love for us in this: While we were still sinners, Christ died for us.*

If my faith is in Christ, God is not waiting to judge and condemn me.

- 1 John 4:16-18, *God is love. Whoever lives in love lives in God, and God in them. This is how love is made complete among us so that we will have confidence on the day of judgment: In this world we are like Jesus. There is no fear in love. But perfect love drives out fear, because fear has to do with punishment. The one who fears is not made perfect in love.*

- Romans 8:1-2, *Therefore, there is now no condemnation for those who are in Christ Jesus, because through Christ Jesus the law of the Spirit who gives life has set you free from the law of sin and death.*

God sees my suffering, cares, and will work on my behalf.

- Jeremiah 14:17, (This is God speaking a direct message through the prophet.) *Let my eyes overflow with tears night and day without ceasing; for the Virgin Daughter, my people, has suffered a grievous wound, a crushing blow.*

- Isaiah 51:3, *The Lord will surely comfort Zion and will look with compassion on all her ruins; he will make her deserts like Eden, her wastelands like the garden of the Lord. Joy and gladness will be found in her, thanksgiving and the sound of singing.*

Appendix C

Steps to Transforming
the Mind

1) Recognize your wrong thinking (repentance/confession).

You know what your wrong thinking is. Admit it in detail to God. Tell him what has brought it about in your thinking and confess that you have in the past chosen to believe these things in place of the truth found in His Word. Admit to Him that you are helpless to change this wrong thinking on your own and ask Him to do the work in you through His Word and Spirit.

2) Focused concentration (meditate day and night on the truth of God's Word).

Find and write down Bible verses that speak the truth about whatever area that you need to dwell on to counter your false views and patterns of thought. Begin to memorize one or two of those passages.

3) Replace the old thoughts with the new (dwell on and quote specific verses so that your mind is renewed and transformed by God's truth).

Every time the old thoughts and fears come to mind, immediately counter them with the Bible verses on which you have been meditating. When you find yourself falling into the old patterns of thought, confess it once again and ask God for help. Then read or quote the Bible verses. Cling to the truth that IN Christ, you are a new creation. The old is GONE, behold all things are made new! (2 Corinthians 5:17)

Appendix D

My Worth IN Christ

I am the righteousness of Christ

- Romans 3:22, **This righteousness is given through faith in Jesus Christ to all who believe.**

- **Romans 4:5, However, to the one who does not work but trusts God who justifies the ungodly, their faith is credited as righteousness.**

- 2 Corinthians 5:21, **God made him who had no sin to be sin for us, so that in him we might become the righteousness of God.**

- Philippians 3:8-10, **that I may gain Christ and be found in him, not having a righteousness of my own that comes from the law, but that which is through faith in Christ--the righteousness that comes from God on the basis of faith.**

I am a new creation in Christ

- 2 Corinthians 5:17, **Therefore, if anyone is in Christ, the new creation has come: The old has gone, the new is here!**

- Colossians 3:3, **For you died, and your life is now hidden with Christ in God.**

I am loved in Christ

- Romans 8:39, **neither height nor depth, nor anything else in all creation, will be able to separate us from the love of God that is in Christ Jesus our Lord.**

- Ephesians 3:17-18, **I pray that out of his glorious riches he may strengthen you with power through his Spirit in your inner being, so that Christ may dwell in your hearts through faith. And I pray that you, being rooted and established in love, may have power together with all the Lord's holy people, to grasp how wide and long and high and deep is the love of Christ**

- Ephesians 5:2, **and walk in the way of love, just as Christ loved us and gave himself up for us as a fragrant offering and sacrifice to God.**

- 1 Timothy 1:14, **The grace of our Lord was poured out on me abundantly, along with the faith and love that are in Christ Jesus.**

I am worthy in Christ

- Ephesians 2:10, **For we are God's handiwork, created in Christ Jesus to do good works, which God prepared in advance for us to do.**

- Ephesians 2:12-13, **Remember that at that time you were separate from Christ, excluded from citizenship in Israel and foreigners to the covenants of the promise, without hope and without God in the world. But now in Christ Jesus you who were once far away have been brought near by the blood of Christ.**

- Colossians 2:9-10, **For in Christ all the fullness of the Deity lives in bodily form, and in Christ you have been brought to fullness.**

I am forgiven in Christ

- Romans 8:1, *Therefore, there is now no condemnation for those who are in Christ Jesus*

- Colossians 1:22, *But now he has reconciled you by Christ's physical body through death to present you holy in his sight, without blemish and free from accusation*

- Romans 8:4, *Who then is the one who condemns? No one. Christ Jesus who died--more than that, who was raised to life--is at the right hand of God and is also interceding for us.*

- 1 Corinthians 6:11, *And that is what some of you were. But you were washed, you were sanctified, you were justified in the name of the Lord Jesus Christ, and by the Spirit of our God.*

- Galatians 2:20, *I have been crucified with Christ and I no longer live, but Christ lives in me. The life I now live in the body, I live by faith in the Son of God, who loved me and gave himself for me.*

Muscle Testing (AK) Explained

Another name for muscle testing is Applied Kinesiology (AK), and there are many variations in how it is done and what it is used for. It is used to test for allergies, to diagnose conditions, to determine emotional baggage, to determine which supplements and how many to take, to determine which materials to use in dental fillings, and even in veterinary care. It also seems to have become an integral part of the thriving market for essential oils. It is everywhere! There are also machines that practitioners sometimes use in place of physical muscle testing, which, in spite of the apparent high-tech gadgetry, is the same thing. Muscle testing proponents say that it is based on the belief that the body knows what it needs. All we have to do is ask it.

Performing the muscle test is quite simple. The belief is that the body gives either a yes or no answer through muscle strength. AK is often used for nutritional or "allergy" testing. In such cases, the individual being tested holds a tiny amount of a suspected allergen or supplement in one hand while extending their other arm to their side at a right angle. The practitioner then places one hand on the individual's shoulder and uses the other hand to lightly press down on the extended arm.

In theory, if allergic to the substance being tested or if the substance would not be good for that individual, the individual's arm muscle will weaken, and the arm can easily be pressed down. If not allergic or the substance would be helpful to the body, the arm remains strong.

It is also possible to self-test using other techniques. Another variation of testing is surrogate testing, which is done through a parent of a young child and in cases where the individual is not capable of performing the strength test themselves. A further method of muscle testing that is practiced by especially "gifted" practitioners is done remotely via phone. In other words, there is absolutely no physical contact with the individual!

For more information on muscle testing, check out the first of three articles in the series "Christians Beware of Muscle Testing" at:

- https://www.heartandmindministries.com/single-post/2016/1/28/None-of-Us-Likes-to-be-Deceived

Or, if you prefer audio, here is a link to "11 Reasons Muscle Testing Is Divination."

- https://www.youtube.com/watch?v=Bs4tg8sJUXg&t=1s

The best resource for understanding concerns with muscle testing, the machines of energy medicine, homeopathy, Rife, frequency medicine, and many other topics within energy medicine is the book, *Ouija Medicine—The Dark Side of Energy Medicine* by Marci Julin.

- https://a.co/d/4QnOkbN

Appendix F

11 Red Flags to Look Out for With Alternative Medical Practices

1. Is the information acquired by the practice the result of secret knowledge?
2. Do you have a sense of unease (lack of peace) with regard to the practice?
3. Have the results of alternative testing been verified through traditionally accepted methods (blood tests, x-rays, etc.) or do the alternative methods contradict traditional results?
4. Does the method used for testing or treatment ever occur through a surrogate, by telephone, or by a machine that has not been scientifically proven to consistently achieve valid results?
5. Is a mysterious gifting required to perform the alternative practice or does the presence of certain people interfere with the effectiveness of the diagnoses or treatment? (i.e. a spouse must leave the room)
6. Are the methods consistent with historically Satanic practices or chance? Are they considered New Age or tied to eastern religions?
7. Do the practices produce "bondage" in people?
8. Do the explanations for how it works use any of the following buzzwords: energy, quantum physics, chi, chakras, the subconscious, inner child, tapping, talk of the body as though it is a separate entity-- "the body knows how to fix itself, the body doesn't lie," frequency, etc.?
9. Anything that uses muscle testing in any form is divination and, therefore, forbidden for the Christian.
10. Over time, does the general progression of symptoms worsen, even though there may be individual improvements? Are the symptoms that develop strange, include suicidal thoughts, or is there great fighting and strife in your home?
11. Have you developed symptoms characterized as Lyme Disease, EMF or mold sensitivity, heavy metal poisoning, parasites, dizziness, or brain fog but have not, through traditionally accepted testing, been shown to have these conditions?

Appendix G

Steps to Repent & Rebuke Evil Spirits

*Submit yourselves, then, to God. Resist the devil, and he will flee
from you. Come near to God and he will come near to you. Wash
your hands, you sinners, and purify your hearts, you double-
minded.* James 4:7-8

1. Submit yourself to God in confession & repentance

Before you do any rebuking of spirits, you must first confess your sin
and tell God of your desire to repent. Ask for his protection and
authority over demons. If your children are old enough to understand,
and they have been a part of it, then explain to them in simple terms
before including them in being present when you follow James 4:7-8.
Even though they are involved at your direction, they may personally
need to repent as well. From my own son and the stories of others, it is
apparent that children are very susceptible to Satan's influence and
spiritual dreams are not uncommon. Make sure they're appropriately
included in your family's repentance.

2. Rebuke the devil out loud in the name of Jesus

Luke 4:35 / Luke 10:17 / Acts 19:13-16

It is clear from passages in the Gospels that the rebuking of evil spirits
was done out loud. It is also clear from the NT that it is only the name
of Jesus that has any authority over Satan. I strongly caution anyone
who is not certain of their salvation (through the blood of Christ alone)
about rebuking Satan. It is Christ's presence indwelling a believer that

allows the individual to have authority over demons, and Acts 19:13-16 tells a story of caution for those who are not saved.

I have heard some teach that you must name the spirits to rebuke them, but this isn't necessary according to almost all instances in the Bible. One other suggestion I have for women: If your husband has also been involved, I encourage you to discuss this with him and ask him as the biblically mandated head of his family to lead your family in rebuking Satan.

3. Eliminate ALL paraphernalia & literature from those practices regardless of the cost.

Acts 19:18-20 says, *Many of those who believed now came and openly confessed what they had done. A number who had practiced sorcery brought their scrolls together and burned them publicly. When they calculated the value of the scrolls, the total came to fifty thousand drachmas. In this way the word of the Lord spread widely and grew in power.*

As I have said, many people have contacted me through my website indicating that they have decided to repent of their involvement with muscle testing, and they have followed James 4:7-8 to do so. However, they stop short of completely eliminating every trace of stuff from that time. It's very hard to give up things that cost a lot of money. However, that is exactly the model we see in Acts 19:18-20. To leave something behind gives the devil a continued foothold in your life and a ground to stand on for temptation. Do not allow this to happen. With repentance comes healing, but repentance means completely turning from that sin. Don't think about it or dwell on it. Just do it!

It can be surprisingly difficult to break free of these practices. If you have questions, need encouragement or support, please feel free to contact me through my website.

https://www.heartandmindministries.com/

Appendix H

Biblical Fasting

Reasons for fasting:

- **To end bondage:** <u>Isaiah 58:6</u>, *"Is not this the kind of fasting I have chosen: to loose the chains of injustice and untie the cords of the yoke, to set the oppressed free and break every yoke?*

  <u>Daniel 9:2-3</u>: *In the first year of his reign, I, Daniel, understood from the Scriptures, according to the word of the LORD given to Jeremiah the prophet, that the desolation of Jerusalem would last seventy years. So I turned to the Lord God and pleaded with him in prayer and petition, in fasting, and in sackcloth and ashes.*

- **For healing:** <u>Isaiah 58:8-9</u>, *Then your light will break forth like the dawn, and your healing will quickly appear; then your righteousness will go before you, and the glory of the LORD will be your rear guard. Then you will call, and the LORD will answer; you will cry for help, and he will say: Here am I.*

  <u>Psalm 35:13</u>, *Yet when they were ill, I put on sackcloth and humbled myself with fasting.*

- **To seek God's intervention:** <u>Esther 4:16</u>, *Go, gather together all the Jews who are in Susa, and fast for me. Do not eat or drink for three days, night or day. I and my attendants will fast as you do. When this is done, I will go to the king, even though it is against the law. And if I perish, I perish."*

  <u>Ezra 8:21</u>, *There, by the Ahava Canal, I proclaimed a fast, so that we might humble ourselves before our God and ask him for a safe journey for us and our children, with all our possessions.*

- **In humble repentance:** <u>Nehemiah 9:1</u>

- **To seek guidance:** <u>Acts 13:2</u> *While they were worshiping the Lord and fasting, the Holy Spirit said, "Set apart for me Barnabas and Saul for the work to which I have called them."*

Instructions for fasting:

- **No fighting or selfish pursuits:** <u>Isaiah 58:3-4</u>, *'Why have we fasted,' they say, 'and you have not seen it? Why have we humbled ourselves, and you have not noticed?' Yet on the day of your fasting, you do as you please and exploit all your workers. Your fasting ends in quarreling and strife, and in striking each other with wicked fists. You cannot fast as you do today and expect your voice to be heard on high.*

- **Do it secretly:** <u>Matthew 6:16-18</u>, *"When you fast, do not look somber as the hypocrites do, for they disfigure their faces to show others they are fasting. Truly I tell you, they have received their reward in full. But when you fast, put oil on your head and wash your face, so that it will not be obvious to others that you are fasting, but only to your Father, who is unseen; and your Father, who sees what is done in secret, will reward you.*

- **Or, with others:** <u>Acts 13:2</u> & <u>14:23</u>, <u>Esther 4:3 &16</u>

The underlying purpose of biblical fasting is to humbly seek God's mercy, which is far more than merely not eating. By denying the demands of the body, we recognize our humble dependance on the LORD. Do you require special mercy in guidance, deliverance, healing, or a repentant heart? Throughout Scripture, we see fasting utilized as a special means for unique situations. It is not a time of punishing oneself for sin or so that God will forgive us (for this we already have upon confession), but so that we might request God's further mercy in light of the consequences of sin.

The time that would have been spent in feeding the flesh is spent instead on seeking God. When I have replaced meals with the bread of heaven (the Lord), I always discover that the struggle with hunger is minimal, unlike when I have fasted for purely physical reasons. Fasting is a spiritual discipline and should be treated as such.

Acknowledgments

During the two years of writing this book, a handful of people have come alongside to make its completion possible. God knew that I could not bear up under the immensity of this endeavor without the encouragement of others, and so, in addition to my husband, He sent me Michelle Johnson, Meg Grimm, and Dawn Rigel.

Michelle, God sent you to me, almost at the start. Though we have yet to meet, you have become a dear friend and sister in Christ. You have faithfully edited, prayed, and cheered me on to the end. It was your encouragement over the last two years that spurred me on countless times. Thank you.

Meg, you came into the picture part way through this project when I desperately wanted to throw in the towel. But, there you were, full of energy, enthusiasm, and much-needed edits, reminding me that I was not in this alone. Thank you.

Dawn, my long-time friend and sister in Christ--Over the past two years, the afternoons spent with you at Panera Bread discussing the chapters I had written always reminded me of the worthwhileness of this endeavor and strengthened me to press on. Your knowledge of biology and functional medicine, combined with your willingness to check my research on medical matters was invaluable. Thank you.

Seth, my wonderful husband--You were stuck endlessly editing my work and listening to me talk through this subject matter for many, many years. You have the patience of Job. For more reasons than one, this book could not have been completed without you. Thank you for generously sharing your time, skill, and keen mind in order to bring this book to completion. You are still my hero.

Finally, thank you, my son, Caleb, for using your graphic design skills to design my book cover.

About the Author

Born in southern California but primarily raised in the Atlanta area, Marci Julin is one of four children. At a young age, she heard the Gospel in a Baptist Sunday school class and responded by placing her trust in Jesus Christ for salvation. At 8 years old she felt the call of God to reach the lost with the Good News of Jesus Christ and had the unique privilege of spending her teenage summers on the mission field. That desire to see people come to saving faith in Jesus Christ never abated, but the realities of life prevented full-time service until she became an empty nester.

While attending Bryan College, a Christian liberal arts college in Dayton, Tennessee, she met Seth, and then married, him in 1991. Before the birth of their son, they moved to the Orlando, Florida area to be near family and continued to reside there for 25 years. Although she graduated from Bryan with a bachelor's degree in elementary education and a minor in Bible, Marci chose to be a homemaker and home-school their only child, Caleb, through the 7th grade. She then taught for two years at her son's classical Christian school.

Despite always feeling God's hand on her life and desiring to please Him, Marci struggled with depression and trusting that God loved her personally due to many years of plaguing health problems. As a type A, driven person she continued pushing herself to her physical limits, always striving to be perfect in everything in order to win the approval of her Lord. It wasn't until God allowed her to become bedridden that she was forced to deal with her misconceptions about God and His deep, unfailing love for her. As the merciful Savior brought healing to her heart and mind through Scripture, He also brought complete physical healing. She now wholeheartedly agrees with the Psalmist when he says, *It was good for me to be afflicted so that I might learn your decrees. The law from your mouth is more precious to me than thousands of pieces of silver and gold* (Psalm 119:71-72).

Since her son, Caleb left home to attend Bryan College, Marci began Heart & Mind Ministries and has devoted her time to biblical teaching, writing, and speaking. Before the birth of Marci's first grandson, God orchestrated their move to beautiful north Georgia where they enjoy being near Caleb and his family. For over ten years Marci and Seth cared for his parents until both left behind the troubled minds of Alzheimer's for their eternal rewards in heaven.

Marci enjoys traveling and exploring the beautiful areas of God's amazing creation, running, gardening, beekeeping, and studying God's Word. Although acutely aware of the sanctifying work that God still needs to accomplish in her, Marci longs to inspire others with a passion for God's Word and a love for her Savior.

- You can gain access to Marci's content or contact her regarding scheduling her for speaking to a women's group on her website at
  https://www.heartandmindministries.com

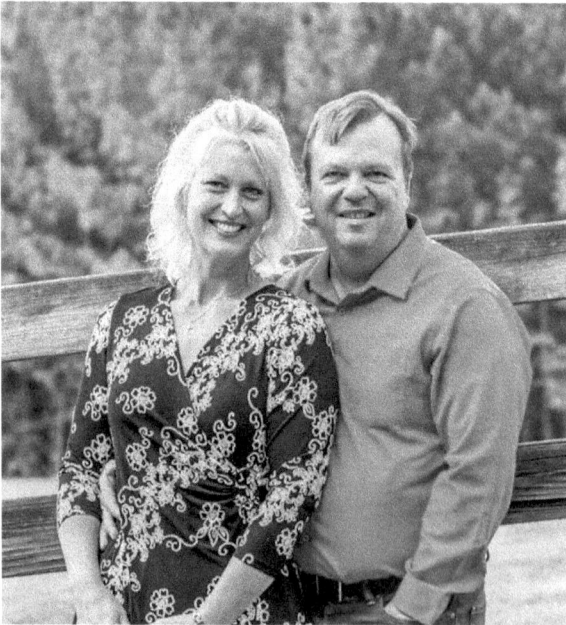

Index

End Notes

[1] Strongs Exhaustive Concordance of the Bible #734.

[2] Strongs Exhaustive Concordance of the Bible #2416

[3] This section is reprinted from When You Can't Trust His Heart-- Discovering the Limitless Love of God, Marci Julin.

[4] http://www.biblestudytools.com/dictionary/heart/ Bruce K. Waltke

[5] Strongs Exhaustive Concordance of the Bible, Hebrew #5315 & Greek # 5590 & #4151.

[6] Strongs Exhaustive Concordance of the Bible, #7307.

[7] The Heart's Code: Tapping the Wisdom and Power of Our Heart Energy, Paul Pearsall, Ph.D.

[8] Biographical Memoirs: Volume 88 (2006), Chapter: John I. Lacey, J. Richard Jennings and Michael G. H. Coles, p230.

[9] American Psychologist, 1977, 1985

[10] ibid

[11] Cameron O. G. (2002). Visceral Sensory Neuroscience: Interoception. New York, NY: Oxford University Press [Google Scholar]

[12] "The Heart, Mind and Spirit" by Professor Mohamed Omar Salem. Murphy et al 2000.

[13] Meda, Karuna, The Heart's "Little Brain", April, 19, 2022, https://research.jefferson.edu/2022-magazine/the-hearts-little-brain.html

[14] ibid

[15] Tiwari R, Kumar R, Malik S, Raj T, Kumar P. Analysis of Heart Rate Variability and Implication of Different Factors on Heart Rate Variability. Curr Cardiol Rev. 2021;17(5):e160721189770. doi: 10.2174/1573403X16999201231203854. PMID: 33390146; PMCID: PMC8950456.

[16] ibid

[17] Pressman, S. D., Gallagher, M. W., & Lopez, S. J. (2013). Is the Emotion-Health Connection a "First-World Problem"? Psychological Science, 24(4), 544-549. https://doi.org/10.1177/0956797612457382

[18] Miller, Michael, MD, "Emotional Rescue: The Heart-Brain Connection," Cerebrum. 2019 May 1;2019:cer-05-19. PMID: 32206169; PMCID: PMC7075501.https://www.ncbi.nlm.nih.gov/pmc/articles/PMC7075501

[19] Yusuf S, Hawken S, Ounpuu S, Dans T, Avezum A, Lanas F, McQueen M, Budaj A, Pais P, Varigos J, Lisheng L; INTERHEART Study Investigators. Effect of potentially modifiable risk factors associated with myocardial infarction in 52 countries (the INTERHEART study): case-control study. Lancet. 2004 Sep 11-17;364(9438):937-52. doi: 10.1016/S0140-6736(04)17018-9. PMID: 15364185.

[20] ibid

[21] Huang, M., et al., Identification of novel catecholaminecontaining cells not associated with sympathetic neurons in cardiac muscle. Circulation, 1995. 92(8(Suppl)): p. I-59.

[22] Cantin, M. and J. Genest, The heart as an endocrine gland. Pharmacol Res Commun, 1988. 20 Suppl 3: p. 1-22.

[23] Vollmar, A.M., et al., A possible linkage of atrial natriuretic peptide to the immune system. Am J Hypertens, 1990. 3(5 Pt 1): p. 408-11.

[24] Johnson, Jon, medically reviewed by Darragh O'Carroll, MD, What Does the Hypothalamus Do?, February 16, 2023, https://www.medicalnewstoday.com/articles/312628

[25] Ocran, Edwin, MBChB, MSc, Hypothalamus, Reviewer: Dimitrios Mytilinaios, MD, PhD, Ken Hub, Last review ed: October 30, 2023, https://www.kenhub.com/en/library/anatomy/hypothalamus

[26] http://www.endocrineweb.com/endocrinology/overview-hypothalamus

[27] Kukanova B, Mravec B. Complex intracardiac nervous system. Bratisl Lek Listy. 2006;107(3):45-51. PMID: 16796123.

[28] Online Etymology Dictionary, from
https://www.etymonline.com/word/disease
[29] Antonovksy, A., *Unraveling The Mystery of Health: How People Manage Stress and Stay Well*. San Francisco: Jossey-Bass, 1987.
[30] http://www.nbcnews.com/health/health-news/one-6-americans-take-antidepressants-other-psychiatric-drugs-n695141
[31] Fawcett, Kirstin, *Why Your Antidepressants Stopped Working – and What to Do About It. How to cope with tachyphylaxis.* May 28, 2015 http://health.usnews.com/
[32] Rama, Swami, "The Real Meaning of Meditation," https://yogainternational.com/article/view/the-real-meaning-of-meditation
[33] Doidge, Norman M.D., The Brain That Changes Itself, p.209.
[34] ibid
[35] ibid
[36] ibid, p.173.
[37] ibid. p.210.
[38] ibid. p.170-172,231,254.
[39] Strongs Exhaustive Concordance of the Bible, #3340.
[40] St. Augustine *Quaestiones in Heptateuchum* 2, 73 (the Heptateuch = the first seven books of the OT Scriptures).
[41] Matthew Henry's Commentary, Leviticus 13:1-17.
[42] ibid.
[43] The Expositor's Bible Commentary p. 582.
[44] Winsam, Willow, August 2017, "Emperor Frankenstein: The Truth Behind Frederick II of Sicily's Sadistic Science Experiments." https://www.historyanswers.co.uk/kings-queens/crusader-queen-sibylla-of-jerusalem-sacrificed-the-holy-city-for-love/
[45] Bakwin, H. (1942). Loneliness in infants. *American Journal of Diseases in Children*, p.32.
[46] van der Horst, F.C.P. & van der Veer, R. Integr. psych. behav. (2008) 42: 325. https://doi.org/10.1007/s12124-008-9071-x
[47] St. Augustine of Hippo, The Confessions, Book I.

[48] https://www.merriam-webster.com/dictionary/punishment

[49] https://www.merriam-webster.com/dictionary/discipline

[50] Strong's Exhaustive Concordance of the Bible, #403.

[51] Strong's Exhaustive Concordance of the Bible, Hebrew #2250 and Greek #3468.

[52] Strong's Exhaustive Concordance of the Bible, Hebrew #2470

[53], Strongs Exhaustive Concordance of the Bible #1321 , Greek *sarx*, Hebrew *besar* #4561.

[54] Doidge, Norman, M.D., The Brain's Way of Healing, p.5.

[55] Melzack, Ronald & Wall, Patrick, "Pain Mechanisms: A New Theory."

[56] Doidge, Norman, M.D., The Brain's Way of Healing, p.5.

[57] Ibid.

[58] Ibid, p.7-9.

[59] Miracles From Heaven, based on a work by Christy Beam, Affirm Films & Columbia Pictures.

[60] "NHS figures show 'shocking' rise in self-harm among young," *The Guardian, October 23, 2016.*

[61] https://www.psychologytoday.com/basics/self-esteem

[62] "Magnetic Resonance Imaging of the Lumbar Spine in People without Back Pain," July 14, 1994, http://www.nejm.org/doi/full/10.1056/NEJM199407143310201

[63] Jensen, Margaret, First We Have Coffee, p.170.

[64] ibid, p.170-171.

[65] Baggoley, C (2015). "Review of the Australian Government Rebate on Natural Therapies for Private Health Insurance". / "Applied Kinesiology". American Cancer Society. *November 2008.* Retrieved August 2013.

[66] Explore (NY). 2014 Mar-Apr;10(2):99-108. doi: 10.1016/j.explore .2013.12.002. Epub 2013 Dec 18. "A double-blind, randomized study to assess the validity of applied kinesiology (AK) as a diagnostic tool and as a nonlocal proximity effect." Schwartz SA1, Utts J2, Spottiswoode SJ3, Shade CW4, Tully L5, Morris WF6, Nachman G7.

[67] Journal of the American Dietetic Association, Kenney JJ, Clemens R, Forsythe KD (June 1988). "Applied kinesiology unreliable for assessing nutrient status". J Am Diet Assoc 88 (6): 698–704. Reprinted in https://en.wikipedia.org/wiki/Applied_kinesiology.

[68] Wurlich, B. (2005), "Unproven techniques in allergy diagnosis". Journal of investigational allergology and clinical immunology 15 (2): 86–90).

[69] Dhakal A, Sbar E. Jarisch Herxheimer Reaction. [Updated 2022 Apr 28]. In: StatPearls [Internet]. Treasure Island (FL): StatPearls Publishing; 2022 Jan-. Available from: https://www.ncbi.nlm.nih.gov/books/NBK557820/ Butler T. The Jarisch-Herxheimer Reaction After Antibiotic Treatment of Spirochetal Infections: A Review of Recent Cases and Our Understanding of Pathogenesis. Am J Trop Med Hyg. 2017 Jan 11;96(1):46-52. doi: 10.4269/ajtmh.16-0434. Epub 2016 Oct 24. PMID: 28077740; PMCID: PMC5239707.

[70] https://www.dhhs.nh.gov/dphs/nhp/documents/sugar.pdf

[71] "Behind New Dietary Guidelines, Better Science," February 2015, Carroll, Aaron E. https://www.nytimes.com/2015/02/24/upshot/behind-new-dietary-guidelines-better-science.html

[72] https://www.thelancet.com/journals/lancet/article/PIIS0140-6736(17)32252-3/fulltext?elsca1=tlxpr

[73] "Associations of egg and cholesterol intakes with carotid intima-media thickness and risk of incident coronary artery disease according to apolipoprotein E phenotype in men: the Kuopio Ischaemic Heart Disease Risk Factor Study," The American Journal of Clinical Nutrition. https://academic.oup.com/ajcn/article/103/3/895/4569580

[74] "Normal-sodium diet compared with low-sodium diet in compensated congestive heart failure: is sodium an old enemy or a new friend?" Clinical Science Jan 08, 2008,114(3)221-230;DOI: 10.1042/CS20070193. http://www.clinsci.org/content/114/3/221

[75] https://www.nytimes.com/2015/02/24/upshot/behind-new-dietary-guidelines-better-science.html

[76] Fallon, Sally. Nourishing Traditions, p.27.

[77] ibid, p.21.

[78] ibid, p.33-34.

[79] ibid, p.38 & 44.

[80] ibid, p.42.

[81] "Transposable Elements: Targets for Early Nutritional Effects on Epigenetic Gene Regulation," Robert A. Waterland, Randy L. Jirtle, Molecular and Cell Biology, https://mcb.asm.org/content/23/15/5293, DOI: 10.1128/MCB.23.15.5293-5300.2003

[82] Johnson, Lorie, "New Science of Epigenetics Proves DNA is not destiny," June 26, 2018, http://www1.cbn.com/cbnnews/health/2018/june/new-science-of-epigenetics-proves-dna-is-not-destiny.

[83] "Epigenetics and male reproduction: The consequences of paternal lifestyle on fertility, embryo development, and children lifetime health." https://www.researchgate.net/publication/283753637_Epigenetics_and _male_reproduction_The_consequences_of_paternal_lifestyle_on_ferti lity_embryo_development_and_children_lifetime_health

[84] Max-Planck-Gesellschaft, "Epigenetics between the generations: We inherit more than just genes." ScienceDaily, July 17, 2017 , from <www.sciencedaily.com/releases/2017/07/170717100548.htm>.

[85] ibid

[86] Sarkar, Fazlul H., editor, Epigenetics and Cancer, p.273.

[87] ibid

[88] "Epigenetics and male reproduction: The consequences of paternal lifestyle on fertility, embryo development, and children lifetime health." https://www.researchgate.net/publication/283753637_Epigenetics_and _male_reproduction_The_consequences_of_paternal_lifestyle_on_ferti lity_embryo_development_and_children_lifetime_health

[89] "A Decade of Exploring the Mammalian Sperm Epigenome: Paternal Epigenetic and Transgenerational Inheritance," Alexandre Champroux, Julie Cocquet, Joëlle Henry-Berger, Joël R. Drevet and Ayhan Kocer, Front. Cell Dev. Biol., May,15 2018, https://doi.org/10.3389/fcell.2018.00050

[90] ibid

[91] "Epigenetics and male reproduction: The consequences of paternal lifestyle on fertility, embryo development, and children lifetime health." https://www.researchgate.net/publication/283753637_Epigenetics_and_male_reproduction_The_consequences_of_paternal_lifestyle_on_fertility_embryo_development_and_children_lifetime_health.

[92] ibid.

[93] Abstract, "Smoking-induced genetic and epigenetic alterations in infertile men," Gunes S1,2, Metin Mahmutoglu A1,Arslan MA1,2, Henkel R3, published in Pubmed, https://www.ncbi.nlm.nih.gov/pubmed/30132931. and "Genetics and epigenetics of alcohol dependence," Vanessa Nieratschker, Anil Batra, and Andreas J Fallgatter, Journal of Molecular Psychiatry 20131:11, https://doi.org/10.1186/2049-9256-1-11.

[94] "In Utero Alcohol Exposure, Epigenetic Changes, and Their Consequences," Michelle Ungerer, Jaysen Knezovich, M.Sc., and Michele Ramsay, Ph.D., Alcohol Res. 2013; 35(1): 37–46. PMCID: PMC3860424, PMID: 24313163, https://www.ncbi.nlm.nih.gov/pmc/articles/PMC3860424/

[9595] Strong's Exhaustive Concordance of the Bible, #5771 avon meaning, "iniquity, guilt, punishment for iniquity."

[96] Geisler, Norman L., "Epigenetics Offers New Solution to Some Long-Standing Theological Problems: Inherited Sin, Christ's Sinlessness, and Generational Curses Can be Explained," 2010 https://normangeisler.com/epigenetics-offers-new-solution-to-some-long-standing-theological-problems-inherited-sin-christs-sinlessness-and-generational-curses-can-be-explained/.

[97] ibid.

[98] "The Famine Ended 70 Years Ago, but Dutch Genes Still Bear Scars," Carl Zimmer, Jan 31, 2018, from https://www.nytimes.com/2018/01/31/science/dutch-famine-genes.html

[99] ibid

[100] ibid

[101] "Transgenerational transmission of hedonic behaviors and metabolic phenotypes induced by maternal overnutrition, " Gitalee Sarker, Rebecca Berrens, Judith von Arx, Pawel Pelczar, Wolf Reik, Christian Wolfrum & Daria Peleg-Raibstein, Translational Psychiatry, volume 8, Article number: 195 (2018), from https://www.nature.com/articles/s41398-018-0243-2

[102] "Epigenetics and male reproduction: The consequences of paternal lifestyle on fertility, embryo development, and children lifetime health," Liborio Stuppia, Marica Franzago, Patrizia Ballerini, Valentina Gatta, and Ivana Antonumcci, Clinical Epigenetics, November 2015, from https://www.researchgate.net/publication/283753637_Epigenetics_and _male_reproduction_The_consequences_of_paternal_lifestyle_on_ferti lity_embryo_development_and_children_lifetime_health

[103] "Transgenerational Effects of Posttraumatic Stress Disorder in Babies of Mothers Exposed to the World Trade Center Attacks during Pregnancy," Rachel Yehuda, Stephanie Mulherin, Engel Sarah R. Brand, Jonathan Seckl, Sue M. Marcus, Gertrud S. Berkowitz, The Journal of Clinical Endocrinology & Metabolism, Volume 90, Issue 7, 1 July 2005, Pages 4115–4118, from https://doi.org/10.1210/jc.2005-0550

[104] "Hereditary trauma: Inheritance of traumas and how they may be mediated, " April 13, 2014, Source: ETH Zurich Summary: "The consequences of traumatic experiences can be passed on from one generation to the next," from https://www.sciencedaily.com/releases/2014/04/140413135953.htm

[105] ibid

[106] Study: "Childhood Trauma Leaves Genetic Scars, Not Just Emotional, " John Schmid, Milwaukee Journal Sentinel, July 23, 2018, from https://reachmd.com/news/study-childhood-trauma-leaves-genetic-scars-not-just-emotional/1618258/

[107] "Grandma's Experiences Leave a Mark on Your Genes, " Dan Hurley, June 25, 2015, from http://discovermagazine.com/2013/may/13-grandmas-experiences-leave-epigenetic-mark-on-your-genes

[108] "Epigenetic regulation of the glucocorticoid receptor in human brain associates with childhood abuse," McGowan PO, Sasaki A, D'Alessio

AC, Dymov S, Labonté B, Szyf M, Turecki G, Meaney MJ, Natural Neuroscience, 2009 Mar;12(3):342-8. doi: 10.1038/nn.2270 from https://www.ncbi.nlm.nih.gov/pubmed/19234457/
[109] "Epigenetic modifications associated with suicide and common mood and anxiety disorders: a systematic review of the literature, " Abdulrahman M El-Sayed, Michelle R Haloossim, Sandro Galea, and

Karestan C Koenen, Biol Mood Anxiety Disord. 2012; 2: 10, Published online 2012 Jun 14. doi: [10.1186/2045-5380-2-10], from https://www.ncbi.nlm.nih.gov/pmc/articles/PMC3495635/
[110] "Differential patterns of whole-genome DNA methylation in institutionalized children and children raised by their biological parents, " Oksana Yu. Naumova, Maria Lee, Roman Koposov, Moshe Szyf, Mary Dozier, and Elena L. Grigorenko, Published online 2011 Nov

29. doi: 10.1017/S0954579411000605, from https://www.ncbi.nlm.nih.gov/pmc/articles/PMC3470853
[111] ibid. Previous studies referred to by the quote I have included: Caldji et al., 2000; Champagne et al., 2003; Franklin et al., 2010; Liu et al., 2000; Meaney & Szyf, 2005; Murgatroyd et al., 2009; Oberlander et al., 2008; Weaver et al., 2004.
[112] "The long-lasting health effects of separating children from their parents at the U.S. border," Melissa Healy, June 20, 2018, The Los Angeles Times, from http://www.latimes.com/science/sciencenow/la-sci-sn-separating-children-psychology-20180620-story.html
[113] ibid
[114] "Differential patterns of whole-genome DNA methylation in institutionalized children and children raised by their biological parents, " Oksana Yu, Naumova, Maria Lee, Roman Koposov, Moshe Szyf, Mary Dozier, and Elena L Grigorenko, Published online 2011 Nov

29. doi: 10.1017/S0954579411000605, from https://www.ncbi.nlm.nih.gov/pmc/articles/PMC3470853/
[115] "Grandma's Experiences Leave a Mark on Your Genes," Dan Hurley, June 25, 2015, from http://discovermagazine.com/2013/may/13-grandmas-experiences-leave-epigenetic-mark-on-your-genes

116 "Hsa-miR-30d, secreted by the human endometrium, is taken up by the pre-implantation embryo and might modify its transcriptome, " Vilella, Moreno-Moya, Balaguer, Grasso, Herrero, Martínez, Marcilla, Simón, 2015 Sep 15;142(18):3210-21. doi: 10.1242/dev.124289, from https://www.ncbi.nlm.nih.gov/pubmed/26395145

117 "Using Donor Eggs? Your Body Is Still Influencing Your Baby's Genes," Rachel Lehmann-Haupt, from http://lehmannhaupt.com/2016/01/06/becoming-a-solo-mom-via-assisted-reproductive-technology-donor-eggs/

118 Nesterak, Evan, The End of Nature Versus Nurture, July 10, 2015, from http://thepsychreport.com/books/the-end-of-nature-versus-nurture/

119 ibid

120 Genetic Science Learning Center. (2013, July 15) "Epigenetics & Inheritance," Retrieved October 18, 2018, from https://learn.genetics.utah.edu/content/epigenetics/inheritance/

121 "Grandma's Experiences Leave a Mark on Your Genes," Dan Hurley, June 25, 2015, from http://discovermagazine.com/2013/may/13-grandmas-experiences-leave-epigenetic-mark-on-your-genes

122 "Epigenetic programming by maternal behavior," Ian C G Weaver, Nadia Cervoni, Frances A Champagne, Ana C D'Alessio, Shakti Sharma, Jonathan R Seckl, Sergiy Dymov, Moshe Szyf & Michael J Meaney, Nature Neuroscience volume7, pages847–854 (2004), from https://www.nature.com/articles/nn1276#abstract

123 "Grandma's Experiences Leave a Mark on Your Genes, " Dan Hurley, June 25, 2015, from http://discovermagazine.com/2013/may/13-grandmas-experiences-leave-epigenetic-mark-on-your-genes

124 Strong's Exhaustive Concordance of the Bible, #7495.

Peace
WITH GOD, SELF, & OTHERS

THE PATH OF LIFE

TRAVELING TOGETHER

A Free Study

Do you need support as you walk this path of life and want to go deeper with God? Consider joining a Path of Life group. Online meetings worldwide.

WWW.HEARTANDMINDMINISTRIES.COM

Question the Narrative

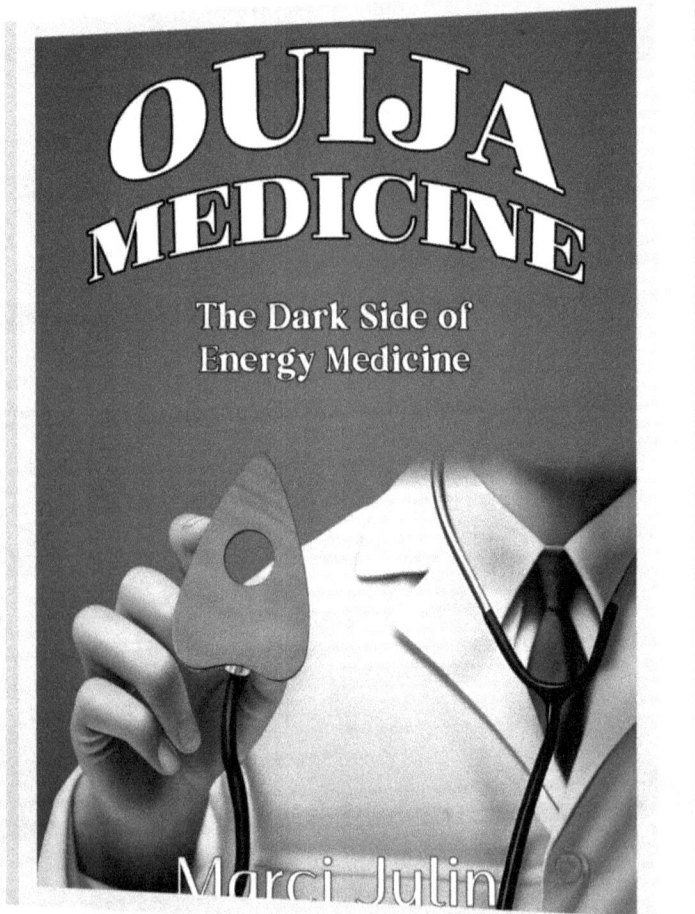

OUIJA MEDICINE
The Dark Side of Energy Medicine

Marci Julin

Available by all booksellers

www.ingramcontent.com/pod-product-compliance
Lightning Source LLC
Chambersburg PA
CBHW070054030426
42335CB00016B/1883